TABL

Printed in Canada

THERESA DALE PH.D., F.A.C.A.C.N.

Director of the Society for Bio-Energetic Research, Speaker, T.V. Host, Researcher, Certified Clinical Nutritionist, Board Certified Naturopathic Medical Doctor

A pioneer in her field for 15 years brings you the latest recipes for your health.

The recipes found in this book will help you to achieve a healthier lifestyle while delighting your palate. You can purchase most items in your local health food store. If they do not carry an item they will order it for you.

Cow milk has been substituted with Soy Milk or Almond/Seed milk. Fertile eggs are in some of the dessert recipes and are optional and substituted where indicated. According to 15 years of my research, I suggest eliminating from your diet all red meat, poultry, shellfish as well as dairy products (cow's or goat's milk products). Other harmful foods are deep fried foods, white sugar, and commercial salt. My clients really excel in health when they eliminate smoking, recreational drugs and alcohol. Not only can you achieve a more healthy, vibrant and energetic body you may also notice people remarking how much younger you look! Remember, daily exercise which includes stretching is crucial to being fit and limber no matter what age you are! Here's to your health!

This cookbook is designed for everyone who is truly interested in longevity and having optimum vitality. Although it has many macrobiotic recipes it also can be used by those who occasionally use eggs in their dietary regime. From my research, I have decided to incorporate the macrobiotic food combining principles as I feel they are the best for most people.

I strongly recommend limited salt and the very occasional usage of eggs in baked goods as well as a limited usage of sweets in the diet.

As each persons health issues are different please take into account what your body needs to function at its optimum level. You will find no red meat, poultry, dairy or refined white sugar in this book as they are not healthy foods for optimum vitality and overall human consumption.

Bon Appetite.

Dr. Theresa Dale, Ph.D.N.D., C.C.N.
Fellow American Council of Applied Clinical Nutrition

1-800-META-404

HERBS AND SPICES

BASIL, fresh or dried, is a versatile herb used in tomato dishes and many others. Be careful with the quantity, as its dominant flavor gets stronger with cooking. Relieves spasms or cramps, excites appetite, expels gas from the intestines, strengthens and stimulates the stomach, helps the body assimilate amino acids.

CAYENNE AND PAPRIKA are great for zesty Mexican dishes, in small amounts adds flavor to bland foods. Excites appetite, stimulates digestive process, stimulant, general invigorator and strengthener. However, cayenne and paprika are irritants: excessive use can cause digestive problems.

CELERY SEED (powdered) is good in soups, stocks, stir fries and more. Its a mild stimulant, expels intestional gas, increases discharge of fluids through urine (diuretic), and its generally an invigorating and strengthening herb.

CINNAMON comes ground or in whole quills or spikes, good in spiced punches, teas and hot fruit drinks, cooked fruit and sweet baked goods. Is warming in the winter time, relieves gas in the intestines, it's a stimulant and antiseptic (impedes growth of some bacteria).

CLOVES are the spicy dried unopened flower of the beautiful tropical evergreen clove tree. Used much like cinnamon in spiced drinks and teas, and in various baked goods. Soothes pain, antiseptic, stimulant, clove tea relieves nausea, intestinal gas and indigestion, stimulates peristalsis (muscular action that propels matter through alimentary canal).

FENNEL SEED has mild licorice flavor, leaves and seeds are good in soup, salads, sauces and are excellent with fish. Whole seeds are added to breads and other baked goods. The medicinal part is the seed: relieves spasms or cramps, excites appetite, stimulates the stomach and aids in digestion, relieves intestinal gas, diuretic, loosens mucous in respiratory passages (expectorant).

GARLIC is a favorite in many dishes. It's more pungent chopped and crushed than it is whole or sliced. It's flavor becomes more mild with cooking. Destroys or expels intestinal worms, relieves spasms or cramps, relieves intestinal gas, diuretic, expectorant (good for coughs and colds), reduces fever, stimulates and aids digestion, regulates liver and gall bladder, beneficial for heart and circulatory system.

GINGER ROOT comes from a beautiful tropical lily. Fresh ginger is best peeled and sliced thin or grated and added to oriental dishes, sauces, salad dressings, stews, fish, baked goods and many other kinds of dishes. Boosts the effectiveness of other herbs, excites appetite, relieves gas and is a stimulant. Promotes cleansing of the system through slightly increased perspiration. Offsets the usual effects of cold.

KELP, while this seaweed doesn't usually grace most spice shelves, and it may be an acquired taste, it is extremely valuable and can be used to good effect in many dishes. It is a salt substitute full of trace minerals and is a gold mine of nutrients.

OREGANO is a wild marjoram. Commonly used in Spanish, Mexican and Italian dishes it is a good seasoning for meats, salad dressing, vegetables and legumes. Use sparingly. Relieves spasms or cramps, calming, soothing effect, relieves gas, expectorant, strengthens and stimulates the stomach, is general good health herb.

MUSTARD SEEDS good for seasoning all kinds of dishes. It is a stimulant and diuretic. Due to its irritant property it is a mild bowel stimulant and gentle purgative.

NUTMEG is the dried kernel from the inner seed of the nutmeg tree. Used in baked goods and other foods. Relieves intestinal gas and is a stimulant. In small quantities nutmeg acts on the stomach to improve appetite and digestion. Caution: use only reasonably small quantities. Excessive amounts can be toxic.

PARSLEY this well known garnish is great for underlining the flavor of foods without dominating. It tones down the odor of strong vegetables like onions. Combines well with other herbs. Expels intestinal gas, diuretic, good for digestion, relieves spasms or cramps. Good general health herb use liberally.

ROSEMARY good on fish and some vegetables like peas and spinach. Has a dominant flavor so use sparingly. Relieves spasms or cramps, stimulant, good for digestive system, promotes liver function, calms and soothes the nerves. Caution: use reasonable amounts, can be toxic in large quantities.

SAGE is a strong herb which tastes more minty when fresh, tends to become bitter tasting with long cooking. Stimulant, relieves spasms or cramps, reduces congestion, expels intestinal gas, general health invigorator.

THYME this strong, dominating flavor is used frequently in French dishes. Aids in digestion of fatty foods. Relieves cramps, expels intestinal gas, good for respiratory passages, expectorant, good tonic for stomach and nerves. Antiseptic and general good health herb.

HERE ARE A FEW POINTS:

Use common sense. For example: if someone has stomach problems, put the helpful herbs in gentle, easy to digest foods rather than hard to digest foods like eggs, spicy foods, and poor food combinations like carbohydrate/protein or fruit/non-fruit combinations.

Be moderate. Don't use spices in unpalatable and inappropriate quantities just to "pack more in there," the activity of most of these herbs is subtle as should be the flavors.

Each spice reacts differently to cooking. Most spice flavors blend into food more during cooking, but they may lose some of their volatile oils and therapeutic value due to the heat. This varies, of course, for every herb, but its a good idea to add a portion of the spices after cooking.

Most herbs work and taste better when used fresh. Some grocery stores carry fresh herbs in the produce section. Or perhaps you can start your own herb garden in your kitchen, its a lot easier than it sounds. Generally, you'll have to use larger quantities of the fresh than you would of the dried herb.

When shopping for spices avoid those marked "pico-waved" or any other euphemism for irradiaton. There are plenty of spices on the market that are not irradiated. Ask the store manager.

Here's a simple way to find out if a spice will taste good in your dish. Take a taste of your dish. Then, while the food is in your mouth, smell the spice you are considering. This will give you a real sense of how well the spice will blend with the flavors already in the dish. Try it, it really works!

REFERENCES:

Lust, John, THE HERB BOOK, Sini Valley, California: Benedict Lust Publishing/Bantam Books, 1983.

Grieves, M. A MODERN HERBAL. New York: Dover Publications, Inc., 1971.

FOOD COMBINING

YIN - EXPANSIVE FORCE

Guidelines to recognizing Yin and acute Yin

Foods that:

*are grown in hot tropical climates
*have a rapid growth rate such as asparagus
*are easily bruised and very perishable
*are grown above ground. The higher above ground the vegetable grows the more Yin. In other words, the height of the vegetable shows Yinness.
*are purple or bluish show very Yin quality such as beets.
*are high in water content. The more water the more Yin.
*are high in potassium. The more potassium content, the more Yin.
*are high in fat such as avocados and bananas are ex-extreme Yin and also are grown in hot climates.
*are very acid are very Yin.

YANG - CONTRACTING FORCE

Guidelines to recognizing Yang and acute Yang

Foods that:

*have more sodium
*are exactly opposite of Yin
*are more alkaline
*have generally warm colors
*are grown down in the earth
*are more compacted, more dry and hearty
*are slower in growth

COOKING AND COMBINING BALANCED MEALS

Here are some simple rules which will help to prepare a digestible, balanced meal for your family.

*Adding fire through cooking lessens Yin and increases Yang proportion of food.
*On the whole the vegetable kingdom is Yin in comparison to the animal kingdom which is Yang.
*If you are cooking a moderate Yin vegetable and want to change to a more Yang property, cook the Yin vegetable for a long time with a little salt.
*Avoid combinations of Yin ingredients with Yin ingredients lacking Yang.
*Avoid Yang ingredients with Yang ingredients lacking Yin.
*Avoid extreme Yin with extreme Yang.
*Avoid eating any extreme by itself.

Herbs are generally Yin (aromatic). Their function within a carnivorous diet is that of balancing Yang (animal food). It is however the less desireable balance of extremes. Used along with vegetarian dietary habits, herbs cause imbalance in the long run, so use them sparingly please.
*Fruit may be combined with sweet varieties of squash such as acorn and butternut.

YIN (EXTREME)

Alcohol
Dairy Products
Refined products including
  Sugar
Chemicals, preservatives,
  etc.
Tomato
Potato
Eggplant
Mushrooms

Asparagus
Rhubarb
Artichoke
Jerusalem artichoke
Spinach
Beets, yams
Herbs

YANG (EXTREME)

Red meat
Eggs
Chicken
Hard cheese
White meat fish is not quite as
  Yang as blue-skinned fish

Shell fish
Ginseng
Jinenjo (Japanese mountain
  yam)
Red-fleshed fish

YIN (MODERATE)

Leafy greens (mustard, kale,
  watercress, collards,
  etc.)
Chinese cabbage
Cabbage
Cauliflower
Broccoli
Squash (butternut,
  buttercup, etc.)
Turnips
Onions
Corn on the cob

Carrots
Parsnips
Sea vegetables
Beans (aduki, chick-pea,
  lentils)
Tempeh
Tofu
All sweeteners
Fruits

YANG (MODERATE)

Buckwheat
Millet
A small amount of fish (white meat) cooked well with
many vegetables in soup vegetables converted by long cooking
and salt.
Seeds
Nuts

Seitan has both Yin and Yang properties because of
cooking. Within the process of its preparation it is cooked with
both soy sauce and salt.

FOODS THAT ARE BALANCED

Brown Rice

FOOD BALANCED SLIGHTLY TOWARDS YIN

Corn-dry
Oats

Wheat
Barley

CONDIMENTS

YIN

Ginger
Scallions
Brown Rice Vinegar

Umeboshi vinegar
Shisho condiment
Fermentation is Yin

YANG

Tekka
Miso
Soy Sauce

Gomasio seasoning - sea salt
& sesame seeds
Salt is very Yang

Umeboshi plum is both YIN and YANG

REAL FOOD SUBSTITUTIONS

OMIT	USE
Aluminum or non-stick surface cookware	Stainless steel or Corningware cookware
Coffee, Chinese Teas, other caffeinated teas	Herb teas, cereal beverages
Commercial peanut butter	Sesame butter, tahini, cashew butter, almond butter. All peanut butter contains volitile oils which are not healthy for the colon.
Salted Nuts	Tamari roasted nuts, raw nuts and seed.
Sulphured dried fruits	Unsulphured dried fruits, without preservatives, preferably organically grown.
Red meat and poultry	Deep sea fish
Snacks	Popcorn, dried fruit and nuts, raw or tamari roasted nuts, fruit, whole wheat or rye crackers, raw vegetables, granola, whole grain baked goods, confections made with healthy ingredients.
Dairy products	Soy cheese, soy milk and soy yogurt, almond milk, sesame cream.

All purpose flour and cake flour	Whole grain flours such as wheat, rye, corn, oat, rice, or whole wheat pastry flour
Boxed cereals - commercial	Granola or whole, flaked, or cracked grains, cooked or raw (soaked)
Cracker or bread crumbs	Whole grain bread crumbs, whole grain flakes, wheat germ, or crackers made with good ingredients
White rice or other refined grains	Brown rice, bulgur wheat, buckwheat, millet, barley
Sugars (Sucrose, dextrose, glucose, brown sugar, "raw" sugar, corn syrup)	Uncooked, unfiltered honey - use 1/2 honey instead of 1 cup sugar, reduce liquid by 1/4 cup. If no liquid in recipe add 3 tbsp. flour 2) PURE maple syrup 3) unsulphured molasses 4) fruit juices and purees 5) Barley malt or rice syrup
Chocolate	Carob powder (3 tbsp. carob plus 2 tbsp. milk = 1 sq. chocolate)
Cocoa	Carob powder - equal amounts
Baking soda	Low sodium baking powder (aluminum free), 2 parts in place of 1 part soda
Baking powder	Low sodium baking powder (aluminum free)
Cornstarch	Whole grain flours,

Salt

Supermarket brands of
  mayonnaise, high in
  saturated fats

Distilled vinegar

Hydrogenated fats and
  shortenings, refined oils

White pasta (spaghetti,
  macaroni, shells,
  noodles)

Soda pop

Herbs which are irradiated
  and which may contain
  preservatives

arrowroot flour

Sea salt, kelp powder,
  vegetable seasonings,
  tamari soy sauce (1/4
  salt = 1 tsp.
  tamari), miso (1/4 tsp. salt
  = 1 1/2 tsp. miso)

Safflower eggless
  mayonnaise

Unfiltered, unpasteurized
  apple cider vinegar,
  brown rice vinegar,
  balsamic vinegar

Unrefined oils, are best
  canola oil lowest in
  saturated fats, soy or
  safflower oil
  margarine

Whole grain pasta's such
  as
  wheat, oat, rice,
  sesame, Jerusalem
  artichoke and Quinoa

Fresh unfiltered fruit
  juices, juices mixed
  with mineral water,
  herb teas

Only herbs which say they
  are non-irradiated
  from your health food
  store.

WHAT TO THROW OUT

1) refined white and brown sugar

2) bleached and unbleached white flour

3) shortenings that are solid at room temperature, including margarine

4) white rice and pastas made with white flour

5) refined table salt

6) any product with preservatives including freshness preservers BHA and BHT

7) Any food containing sugar, including fruits canned in heavy syrup

8) packaged dry cereals from supermarkets including supermarket granola

9) Hydrogenated peanut butter

10) All synthetic sweeteners and anything made with them

11) Candies and commercial breads that use emulsifiers and preservatives

12) chocolate - 40% white sugar is added to produce sweet chocolate people are used to. Contains theobromine plus caffeine - 2 stimulants. Contains oxalic acid which interferes with calcium absorption.

13) cooking oils, supermarket brands, refined, deodorized, bleached oils

COOKING CHART FOR GRAINS

1 cup of grain:	Amount of boiling water:	Time:
Barley	2 1/2 cups	45 - 60 minutes
Millet	1 3/4 cups	20 minutes
Oat flakes	2 1/2 cups	20 - 30 minutes
Rice, short grain	2 1/2 cups	45 minutes
long grain	1 1/2 cups	45 minutes
flaked	2 cups	20 minutes
Rye, whole	2 1/2 cups	50 - 60 minutes
flaked	2 cups	20 minutes
Wheat, whole	2 1/2 cups	45 - 60 minutes
flaked	2 cups	20 minutes
cracked	3 cups	20 minutes

COOKING TIPS:

Always add grains to boiling water, stir once, cover pan and simmer until cooking time is almost up. To check to see if they're done, put top end of wooden spoon into the middle of the pan and see if water is evaporated. Do not stir, but carefully lift a few grains out of pan and test for tenderness. If done to desired tenderness and there's still water in bottom of pan, remove cover and cook a few more minutes. If not done and there's no water left, add a little more water.

VARIATIONS:

For millet and rice, substitute 1/2 cup Very Vegie Juice (by Knudson) for 1/2 cup water. Or try sauteeing millet or rice in 1 tbsp. unrefined oil with a little minced garlic for about 2 minutes, then add boiling water.

COOKING CHART FOR BEANS

1 cup dry beans:	Soaking time and amount of water:	Time:
Azuki	1 hour (4 cups water)	60 minutes
Black	Overnight (4 cups water)	2 to 3 hours
Chick-peas (Garbonzos)	Overnight (4 cups water)	2 to 3 hours
Kidneys	1 hour (3 cups water)	60 minutes
Lentils	1 hour (3 cups water)	45 minutes
Navy beans	1 hour (3 cups water)	60 minutes
Soy beans	Overnight (4 cups water)	2 to 3 hours
Soy beans, flaked	Unsoaked (2 cups water)	60 to 90 minutes
Split peas	Unsoaked (3 cups water)	45 minutes

NOTE: One cup dry beans makes approximately 2 1/2 cups cooked beans.

Variations: For any bean, add 1 chopped onion, 2 or 3 cloves minced garlic, bay leaf, 1/2 tsp. cayenne pepper, 1 tsp. each of oregano and basil, 1/4 tsp. marjoram. For spicy style, also add 1 tbsp. chili powder, 1 tbsp. cumin, and more cayenne to taste.

KEEPING FOOD FRESH

FOOD	PREFERRED STORAGE TEMP.	RECOMMENDED STORAGE CONDITIONS
Vegetables (most varieties)	Refrigerator	Surface dirt removed, but unwashed; in crisper, storage bags or covered container (7 days)
Mushrooms	Refrigerator	Loosely wrapped (5 to 7 days)
Avocadoes	Ripen at room temp.	Refrigerate when ripe; once cut, bathe surface in lemon juice and leave pit intact to prevent browning (3 to 5 days)
Potatoes, onion, garlic, winter squash	Cold Spot	Dry in ventilated container away from light (1 to 4 weeks)
Sprouts	Refrigerator	Well drained, covered container (5 days)
Fruits (most varieties)	Ripen at room temp; refrigerate when ripe	Thoroughly dried if washed in crisper (5 to 7 days)

Milk/Cream	Refrigerator	
		Closed, preferably in original or opaque container (7 days)
Yogurt, Sour cream	Refrigerator	
		Closed container (2 weeks)
Eggs	Refrigerator	
		Surface dirt removed, unwashed, covered (2 weeks)
Fish	Refrigerator	
	Freezer	Loosely wrapped (3 to 5 days) Airtight package (3 to 6 months)
Tofu	Refrigerator	
		Submerged in fresh water, changed daily (5 to 7 days), if slightly soured refresh by simmering in water for 10 minutes.
Bread, rolls	Refrigerator	
	Freezer	Tightly wrapped (3-7 days) Airtight wrapper (3-6 months)
Oils	Refrigerator	
		Opaque or closed container in dark spot; harmless clouding may occur.

Food	Storage	Notes
Honey, molasses, maple syrup	Refrigerator	Covered container; gentle heating will reverse granulation. Variable life span.
Nuts and seeds	Below 68 F Room temp	6 to 12 months Airtight container (4 weeks)
	Refrigerator	Airtight container (6 months)
	Freezer	Airtight container (1 year)
Nut Butter	Refrigerator	Up to 6 months
Whole Grains	Below 68 F.	Airtight container (6 to 9 months)
Flours	Refrigerator	Airtight container (6 months)
Pasta (fresh)	Refrigerator	Covered (1 to 2 days)
Herbs	Cold Spot	Airtight container out of direct light (6 months)
Spices (unground) (Ground)	Cold Spot	Airtight container (1 to 2 years)
	Cold Spot	Airtight container out of direct light (6 months)

S o u p S

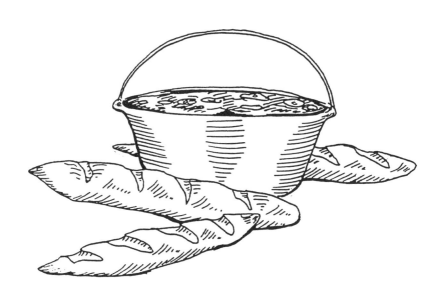

ZUCCHINI-SPLIT PEA SOUP

1/2 onion, chopped
1 to 2 cloves garlic, minced
3/4 c. green split peas
1 bay leaf
6 c. vegetable stock
6 c. diced zucchini

2 tbsp. mixed chopped
  herbs, fresh basil,
  thyme, etc. (or 2 tsp.
  dried herbs)
2 tsp. tamari
1/2 lb. spinach or other
  greens
1/4 c. chopped parsley
1 sm. lemon, sliced thin

Place onion, garlic, split peas and bay leaf in a saucepan with 4 cups of stock. Bring to a boil, then cover and simmer for 40 minutes. Add zucchini, remaining stock and herbs. Cook for another 10 minutes. Remove bay leaf. Puree soup in a blender in batches. Return to the soup pot. Add tamari and adjust herbs if needed. Stir in the spinach or greens and the parsley and cook a few minutes more. Garnish each serving with a thin slice of lemon. This soup may also be served cold.

LENTIL VEGETABLE SOUP

2 c. lentils, washed
8 c. water or vegetable stock
1 onion, chopped
2 cloves garlic, minced
2 lg. celery ribs, chopped

2 lg. carrots, chopped
1 zucchini, chopped
1 tbsp. parsley
2 1/2 tsp. salt
1 slice fresh ginger

Combine the above ingredients in a large soup pot with a cover and bring to a boil. Reduce heat and simmer, covered, for 1 1/2 to 2 hours. Before serving, top with sliced green onions.

SPICY CREAM OF CARROT SOUP

1 tbsp. soy margarine
1 onion, chopped
2 cloves garlic, minced
1/2 tsp. mustard seeds
1/2 tsp. turmeric
1 tbsp. fresh grated ginger
1/2 tsp. ground cumin
1/8 tsp. cayenne pepper

1 lb. carrots, scrubbed and
   sliced 1/2 inch thick
1 tbsp. lemon juice
3 1/2 c. water
1 1/2 c. plain yogurt (soy)
1 tbsp. barley-malt syrup
Miso, to taste, or 1 to 2
   tbsp. light miso
10 oz. cooked green peas
   (optional)
2 tbsp. chopped fresh
   cilantro

    Melt the margarine in a large skillet and saute onion and garlic until they are clear. Add the spices and cook for several minutes, stirring continuously. Add the carrots and lemon juice and cook a few more minutes, still stirring. Add 2 cups of the water, cover and simmer 30 minutes or until carrots are tender. Puree mixture in a blender or food processor with the remaining 1 1/2 cups of water; they may need to be done in batches. Pour puree into a saucepan and whisk in the yogurt and barley-malt syrup. Reheat soup gently; do not allow to boil. Add cooked peas, if desired, and miso (creamed in a cup with a little of the soup). Serve hot or chilled, garnished with a sprinkle of chopped cilantro.

VEGETABLE BARLEY SOUP

1/2 c. diced onion
1/2 c. celery
1/2 c. carrot
1/2 c. bell pepper
2 tbsp. Canola oil

3 c. vegetable stock or
   water
1 c. cooked barley
1/2 tsp. Miso
1/2 c. cabbage, chopped
2 tbsp. chopped scallions

    Saute onion, celery, carrot and bell pepper in Canola oil for about 5 minutes. Add vegetable stock or water, barley, Miso and cabbage and cook about 40 minutes, covered. Add parsley, correct seasonings and serve or refrigerate. This soup is better the second day.

FRESH CORN SOUP

2 sm. ears or fresh corn
4 c. water
2 tsp. oil "Canola"
1 c. chopped onion
1/3 c. cornmeal
1/2 c. chopped celery

Tamari, to taste
1 c. cubed tofu, optional
Garnish: 1/2 c. chopped
green onions or
watercress

Clean corn and remove kernels from the corn cobs gently in 4 cups of water for 7 minutes; save the cooking water.

In another saucepan, saute chopped onion and corn kernels in the oil with Tamari until the onion is clear. Add cornmeal to the vegetables and mix in well. Slowly add reserved cooking water to the pot, stirring constantly to make a creamy, smooth mixture. Bring to a boil. Lower heat and simmer 20 minutes, stirring occasionally. Add a little more water if soup becomes too thick. Add celery and cook 15 minutes longer. Add tamari to taste and cubed tofu, if desired. Serve hot, garnished with chopped green onions or watercress.

POTATO ONION POTAGE

4 onions, sliced very thin
2 lg. potatoes, also thinly
   sliced
2 tbsp. olive oil
2 tbsp. butter "soy"

2 c. soy milk
1/4 c. dark miso
Cayenne pepper to taste

Saute onions and potatoes in oil and butter. Keep heat low and allow potatoes and onion to cook together for 3 hours, stirring at intervals.

Add soy milk; when warm, remove a bit of the milk and cream miso in it. Return miso-milk mixture to the pot, and bring soup just to the boil. Serve immediately, or refrigerate overnight and serve the next day.

BEAN AND BARLEY SOUP

1 1/2 c. azuki beans
1 1/2 c. whole barley
6 to 8 c. water
1 onion, chopped
2 cloves garlic, minced
1 c. diced carrot

1 c. diced celery
2 c. chopped collard greens
3 to 4 tbsp. dark miso
1 tsp. tamari
Vegie salt to taste

In a large pot combine azuki beans and barley. Cover with water. Bring to a rolling boil and add chopped vegetables except the collard greens. Cook until all is tender (about 1 to 1 1/2 hours) and remove from heat and add collard greens. When greens are wilted by the heat, add the miso creamed in a bit of the soup. Season to taste.

ITALIAN VEGETABLE SOUP

1 c. dried white beans, or a combination of dried beans
3 qts. vegetable stock or water
Miso and cayenne pepper to taste
1 sm. head of cabbage, sliced thin
4 to 5 med. carrots, sliced 1/4 inch
1 lb. fresh tomatoes, chopped
1 c. cubed dicon radish

2 onions, sliced
1/4 c. olive oil
2 stalks celery, sliced
2 lg. zucchini, sliced
1 clove garlic, minced
1/2 c. parsley
1 bay leaf
1/2 c. brown rice

Place the beans in a large bowl and add water to cover by 1 inch. soak overnight. Drain and empty into a large soup kettle. Add the stock or water and bring to a boil. Reduce heat, cover and allow to simmer for 1 hour. Add the tomatoes, radish, cabbage and carrots. Allow to simmer covered 30 minutes.
Heat the olive oil in a skillet and gently saute the onions until wilted. Then add the celery, zucchini, garlic and fresh tomatoes. Simmer 20 minutes and then add the parsley. Add to the bean mixture with the rice. Cook until the rice is tender.

CHILLED CUCUMBER SOUP

1 lg. cucumber, peeled and seeded
2 c. plain yogurt (soy)
2 tbsp. lemon juice
2 tsp. fresh chopped dill weed (or 1 tsp. dried)

1 green onion, chopped
2 tsp. olive oil, optional
Tamari and cayenne pepper to taste
2 tbsp. chopped fresh mint

Seed peeled cucumber by halving lengthwise, then running a sharp teaspoon along the center of each half. Chop up one cucumber half and place in a blender or food processor with 1 cup yogurt, the lemon juice, dill weed and green onion. Blend until smooth. shred or finely chop the cucumber half. Combine this in a mixing bowl with the blended mixture, olive oil and the remaining yogurt. Add Tamari and pepper to taste. Chill well. Add a little water if soup is too thick. Garnish with chipped fresh mint.

GAZPACHO

2 lg. tomatoes, quartered
1 med. cucumber, peeled
    and chopped
1 med. green pepper, seeded
    and quartered
2 green onions, chopped
1 clove garlic, crushed
2 sprigs fresh parsley,
    chopped
1 tbsp. chopped fresh basil
    (or 1 tsp. dried)

1 1/2 c. tomato juice
1 tbsp. wine vinegar
1 tbsp. olive oil
2 to 4 tbsp. lemon juice
Dash cayenne pepper or
    hot sauce
1 c. whole wheat bread
    cubes
1 c. cubed tofu
2 tbsp. fresh parsley,
    chopped

This soup may be made in a blender or food processor. If you want to skin the tomatoes, immurse them in boiling water for one minute, then rinse in cool water and slip off the skins. Reserving 1/2 cup of chopped cucumber and 1 chopped green onion for garnish, process the first ten ingredients in a blender or food processor. Pour into a bowl and add next three ingredients, to taste. cover and chill several hours. Add a few ice cubes if your time is limited. When ready to serve, sprinkle reserved chopped green onion and cucumber onto each serving, along with tofu and chopped parsley. Pass the bread cubes in a bowl.

SALMON BISQUE SOUP

1/2 c. soy milk
1 med. head of cauliflower
   or 3 med. white potatoes
2 salmon steaks, deboned
1 tbsp. chopped fresh dill
   weed
2 sm. cloves of garlic,
   minced
2 to 3 med. long green
   onions, chopped
1 tsp. fresh basil, finely
   chopped

4 tbsp. fresh lemon juice
1/2 c. sesame tahini
1 1/2 c. of vegetables stock
   or a dilution of carrot
   concentrate and spring
   or
distilled water
1/2 tsp. sea salt or 1 tsp.
   Miso

First steam the cauliflower or boil the potatoes until soft. At the same time poach the salmon steaks on top of the stove in a covered pan with 1/2 cup distilled water. In a blender: Put chopped cauliflower pieces or potatoes; vegetable stock or carrot concentrate diluted with water and the soy milk. Blend these until smooth.

Now add the deboned salmon, the garlic, lemon juice and tahini and blend until smooth. Pour the ingredients from the blender into a saucepan and add the onions, dill and basil. Heat on top of the stove for about 10 to 15 minutes. The longer you cook, the thicker the consistency. Season to taste.

SUMMER FRUIT DESSERT SOUP

2 tsp. arrowroot
1 tbsp. lemon juice
1 1/4 c. water
2 tsp. barley malt

1 stick cinnamon
8 whole cloves
2 1/2 to 3 c. fresh fruit cut
   in bite size pieces

In saucepan mix together the arrowroot and lemon juice until smooth. Stir in water, barley malt, cloves and cinnamon stick. Stirring constantly, bring mixture to a boil. Reduce heat to simmer and, still stirring constantly, cook five minutes longer to blend flavors. Remove from heat; discard cinnamon stick and cloves. Stir in fruit. Chill. Serves 3 to 4.

Salad Dressings & Gravy

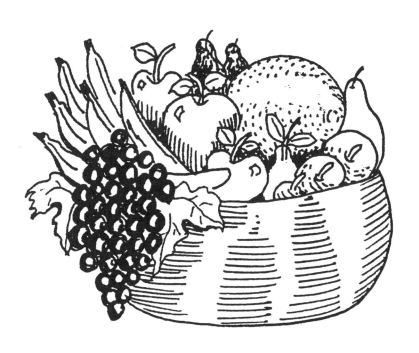

MELON FRUIT CUP

Juice of 1 lg. lemon
1 tbsp. honey
2 med. oranges, sectioned
1 1/2 c. diced cantaloupe

1 1/2 c. white seedless
    grapes or other grapes
    cut in half and seeds
    removed
Fresh mint leaves, optional

Mix the lemon juice and honey until blended. Add fruit and toss gently until fruit is well coated with lemon juice mixture. Chill well. Serve garnished with mint leaves, if desired. Serves 4 to 6.

MELON AU GINGEMBRE

1 big honeydew melon
3 tbsp. lemon or lime juice

1/4 tsp. powdered ginger
    or grated fresh ginger
1 tbsp. honey

Mix the lemon juice, the ginger and honey. Dice the melon and pour the sauce on it. Let it marinate at least 1 hour in the refrigerator before serving.

MELON BOWL SALAD

Wash cantaloupe; cut in half and scoop out seeds. Cut melon out of shells with a melon baller. In a bowl, combine melon balls with other fresh fruits such as blueberries, raspberries, blackberries, seedless grapes, pitted sweet cherries, or sliced strawberries, peaches, nectarines, apricots or plums.

Cut small piece from bottom of cantaloupe shells to make them sit level. Heap fruit mixture into shells and serve plain or topped with favorite fruit salad dressing. Allow 1 filled cantaloupe half per serving.

FENNEL STICKS

Slice one large fennel bulb into sticks, similar to celery sticks. Serve on a small plate after dinner to clear the palate before dessert. Fennel aids digestion, too.

BROCCOLI SALAD

1 1/2 lbs. fresh broccoli
3 hard boiled eggs
2 tbsp. minced onions

1/8 c. mayonnaise
Cayenne pepper and
Tamari to taste

Boil broccoli in salt water until tender. Chop eggs finely and toss with onions and broccoli. Mix mayonnaise with broccoli and season. Chill. This salad will be a favorite to even broccoli haters!

GUACAMOLE

3 ripe avocados
1 chopped onion, chopped
   very fine
1/4 tsp. garlic powder
1/2 tsp. cumin
1/4 tsp. cayenne pepper

1/2 tsp. corriander
1/2 tsp. Indo seasoning
1 chopped tomato
1/2 can black olives,
   chopped
2 tbsp. natural picante
   sauce

Mash all ingredients together and chill for 10 minutes. Leave pit in middle of bowl before serving to prevent guacamole from turning brown.

NOUILLES "SAUCE AUX NOIX"

1 c. chopped fresh parsley
1 tsp. fresh basil
1 tsp. salt or Tamari
1/8 tsp. cayenne pepper, add
   after cooking
3 cloves garlic, minced

1/2 lb. rice or Jerusalem
   artichoke noodles
1/2 c. olive oil
2 tbsp. boiling water
1/4 c. chopped walnuts or
   pine nuts

Cook the noodles. Blend all the other ingredients with a fork or in a food processor or blender. Pour on the hot, drained noodles, toss and serve. This dish can be frozen or kept for some days in the refrigerator.

MISO VEGETABLE TOPPING

Saute:
**1 to 2 c. diagonally sliced
 vegetables
 (cabbage is a good choice)**

In:
1 to 2 tbsp. sesame oil

Add:
**1 tbsp. dark miso (or more
 to taste) and 1 tsp.
 honey or barley malt
sweetener**

Cook, stirring constantly, until vegetables are evenly coated. Cool before serving and store refrigerated or make a double batch and add to it:
4 c. cooked brown rice

In this case, serve hot, garnished with toasted sesame seeds.

TOFU PARTY DIP

2 blocks tofu
6 minced scallions
3 tsp. umabushi plum paste

1 tsp. cayenne pepper
1 minced green pepper

Mash all ingredients together or put in blender on low until creamy consistency. Add sea salt or Tamari to taste.

DEVILED TOFU

Mustard dominates this pungent spread.

8 oz. tofu
**2 tsp. prepared Dijon style
 mustard**
1/2 tsp. tamari
1/8 tsp. turmeric for color
1/4 c. minced green pepper

**1/4 c. minced onion,
 optional**
1/8 tsp. paprika

Mash tofu with fork until crumbly. Add remaining ingredients, except paprika, and mix well. Sprinkle paprika on top. Makes 1 1/2 cups - 3 sandwiches or hors d'oeuvres for 4 to 6.

SPECIAL SPROUT SPREAD

1 c. alfalfa, cabbage, clover
  or radish sprouts
1/2 c. mung bean sprouts
1/2 c. sprouted wheatberries

3 tbsp. vegetable oil
1 to 2 tbsp. lemon juice
1/8 tsp. gomasio seasoning
Sea salt to taste

Grind first 3 ingredients. Blend in the next 4 ingredients. Refrigerate until ready to serve. This is a good basic spread that can be made ahead and kept in the refrigerator up to a week. Add mashed tofu or more oil and it can be used as a dip.

EGGLESS SOY MAYONNAISE

1 c. rich soy milk
4 tsp. honey or rice syrup
1 to 1 1/2 c. safflower oil

1/4 c. lemon juice
1/2 tsp. sea salt
1/4 tsp. cayenne pepper

Blend first 2 ingredients on a low speed, gradually adding oil until it whips up and no longer agitates. Scoop into a bowl and whip in (with a fork or whisk) the next two ingredients, adding gradually. Mixture will stiffen. Add last two ingredients. Mix well and chill. Serve just like mayonnaise.

CASHEW GRAVY

Thick and rich with plain, homey taste. Ideal for grain loaves, burgers and vegetable loaves.

6 tbsp. unroasted cashews
1 1/4 to 1 1/2 cups water
1 tbsp. arrowroot

1 tsp. white miso
Lemon juice

Grind nuts to a powder in a blender or processor. Gradually blend in 1 1/4 cups water to make a smooth "milk".

POPPY SEED - TOFU DIP

1/2 lb. tofu
2 tbsp. tahini
2 tbsp. miso, shiro or kome
2 tbsp. vinegar or lemon
   juice

1/4 to 1/2 c. water
2 tbsp. poppy seeds
2 tbsp. chopped parsley

Mash tofu with fork. Roast tahini in skillet for 2 to 3 minutes. Mix tofu, tahini, miso, vinegar and water in blender. Roast poppy seeds in skillet; stir to prevent burning. When seeds smell nutty, add to tofu mixture in blender. Chop parsley, add to dip, adjust seasonings.

GINGER ASPARAGUS SALAD

This is a very spicy warm salad made with steamed slivers of fresh asparagus and lots of ginger and garlic.

1 lb. asparagus, tough ends
   removed
6 cloves garlic, minced
1 inch gingerroot, grated,
   unpeeled
1/2 tsp. honey

2 tbsp. tamari
2 tsp. sesame oil
1 tbsp. rice vinegar
1 1/2 tsp. hot Szechwan
   peppers, or cayenne

Slice the asparagus into matchsticks by cutting each stalk into 3 inch lengths, then slivering the lengths into thin strips with a sharp paring knife. Steam asparagus for 5 minutes or until crisp tender. Toss warm asparagus with remaining ingredients and serve at room temperature. Serves 4.

PEACH COCONUT SALAD

2 tbsp. lemon juice
2 tbsp. water
1/4 tsp. almond extract
3 c. fresh cubed, unpeeled
   peaches
1/2 c. chopped, pitted dates

1/2 c. broken pecans
1/2 c. shredded,
   unsweetened coconut
1/4 c. yogurt (soy yogurt
   as alternative)
2 tbsp. honey

Mix together the lemon juice, water and almond extract. Add peaches and toss until all cut sides of peaches are coated with lemon juice mixture. Add dates, pecans and coconut.

Mix together the yogurt and honey until smooth and fold gently into fruit mixture. Chill well before serving. Serves 6 to 8.

FRESH PINEAPPLE MOLD

1 1/2 c. fresh pineapple, cut
   into small pieces
1 c. water
1/2 c. apricot nectar juice

4 tbsp. agar flakes
3 mandarin oranges,
   sectioned
1 bananas, sliced

Puree pineapple and water together in a blender. Pour into a saucepan, add apricot nectar and agar, and bring to a boil. Reduce heat and simmer 5 minutes, stirring occasionally. Remove from heat and pour agar mixture into a mold prerinsed with cold water, and refrigerate until it starts to set, about 20 minutes. When agar mixture is ready, gently fold in mandarin oranges and sliced banana. Refrigerate until set. Unmold and garnish with fresh pineapple pieces.

APRICOT SAUCE

2 c. apricot nectar (apricot
   juice in a jar)

1/2 c. dried unsulphured
   apricots, cut into small
   pieces

In saucepan, combine nectar and apricots. Cover and simmer 20 to 25 minutes or until apricots are tender. Chill.

TOMATO-ZUCCHINI SALAD WITH FOURTH-OF-JULY DRESSING

This is a salad to make when you take a basket of extra tomatoes and zucchini to a friend and find that she has a basket of them for you!

3 (6 inch) zucchini, sliced
   thin with skins left on
2 lg. ripe tomatoes, chopped
   coarsely

1 sm. sweet onion, cut in
   rings

Combine vegetables in large glass or crockery bowl. Pour dressing over and toss. Serve immediately.

FOURTH OF JULY DRESSING:

2 tsp. brown rice miso
1/4 c. red wine vinegar
2 tbsp. lemon juice
1 sm. clove garlic, crushed
    in a press
Freshly ground pepper, no
    salt

Dash of each dry mustard,
    paprika, oregano
2 tsp. fresh basil
2/3 c. olive oil

Mix vinegar and lemon juice. Add garlic and spices and mix or shake well. Add oil and stir or shake until dressing is well blended.

LEMON-HERB DRESSING

1 tbsp. honey
5 tbsp. fresh lemon juice
3 tbsp. apple cider vinegar
1 sm. clove garlic, crushed
    in a press

Dried basil and oregano
Fresh cayenne pepper, no
    salt
2/3 c. safflower or very
    mild olive oil

Pour honey into the bottom of a medium sized jar. Add the lemon juice and vinegar and stir until honey is dissolved. Add the seasonings and the oil, cap the jar, and shake well until all ingredients are blended.

To use fresh herbs: substitute 2 medium sized fresh basil leaves, finely chopped for the dried basil. In place of dried oregano, add two large sprigs (about 1 1/2 inches long) summer savory, finely minced. Add two tablespoons chopped chives. Make fresh herb dressing about an hour ahead so that flavors may blend. Fresh herbs are preferred for all cooking needs.

GAZPACHO

A spanish salad you can drink!

1 sm. onion, chopped
1 bell pepper, as ripe as
    possible, chopped (not
    seeded)
1 lg. cucumber, chopped
    (reserve a few slices for
    garnish)
3 ripe tomatoes, about 1 1/2
    lbs., peeled and
    chopped*

2 cloves of garlic, chopped
1/4 c. cider vinegar
2 tsp. sweet paprika
2 tbsp. olive oil (or other
    unrefined vegetable
    oil)
1.8 tsp. cayenne pepper

Blend all ingredients to a smooth puree a little at a time, blending in the vinegar, paprika and oil. Place the puree in a glass or ceramic bowl, and mix very well. Chill. Garnish with the cucumber slices and serve cold. Gazpacho is best when made a day in advance.
    *Peel ripe tomatoes by dropping them in boiling water for 10 seconds. Drain. Rinse. Remove stem end and slip off the skin.

CARROT SALAD

Yield 6 1/2 cup servings.

2 1/2 c. grated carrots
5 tbsp. flaked coconut
5 tbsp. sunflower seeds
5 tbsp. raisins, unsulphered

1/4 lb. tofu
1 1/2 tbsp. safflower oil
1/3 tsp. cinnamon
4 1/2 tsp. cashews

Blend the tofu, oil, cinnamon and cashews until smooth. Mix into carrots, sees, raisins and coconut. Place a few leaves of lettuce on plate, a slice of fresh cored pineapple to the left side of plate and carrot salad to the right, overlapping the pineapple.

SALSA VERDE

Uncooked Green salce. If you can find fresh tomatillos, by all means use them for this salsa. But do not substitute American green tomatoes. The flavor will be quite different.

1 (13 oz.) jar Mexican green tomatoes (tomatillos)
1/4 c. chopped white onions
1 chili, roasted, peeled and seeded
1 tbsp. olive oil

1 tbsp. white wine vinegar
1 tsp. minced garlic
1/4 tsp. sea salt
1/4 tsp. cayenne pepper

Combine tomatoes, onions, chili and puree in blender. Combine with remaining ingredients. Yield: 1 3/4 cups.

KIWIFRUIT TOFU SALAD FOR TWO

1 1/2 c. frozen tofu cubes, thawed and squeezed
1/4 c. chopped celery
1 tbsp. minced scallion
1/4 c. coarsely chopped walnuts

3 tbsp. mayonnaise (natural type made from safflower oil)
Dash tamari
1 kiwifruit, pared and sliced
Lettuce, as needed

Combine tofu with a dash of tamari and remaining ingredients, except lettuce and kiwifruit. Spoon onto two lettuce-lined salad plates. Garnish each serving with kiwifruit slices. Serves 2.

MOUSSE AUX FRUITS

Light as a cloud. Try it with bananas, peaches, apples, apricots or prunes. If you prefer, you can also cook the mousse; pour it in a buttered mold and put it in a 325 degree oven until it sets (30 to 40 minutes), then chill.

2 c. pureed fruits
2 tbsp. lemon juice
4 egg whites

1/2 tsp. cream of tartar
1/4 c. honey or maple syrup

Mix the pureed fruit with the lemon juice. Beat the egg whites until they thicken; add the cream of tartar and drizzle in the honey or syrup and continue to beat until they get medium-stiff. Very carefully, fold the puree into the meringue with a spatula. Garnish with fresh fruits. Try to make this mousse just before serving; it's best when freshly made.

HERBED POTATO SALAD

4 or 5 red boiling potatoes	1 sm. sweet onion,
1/2 c. celery, chopped	chopped
	1/4 c. chopped green
	pepper

HERB DRESSING:

1 tsp. honey	1 lg. fresh basil leaf,
2 tbsp. apple cider vinegar	minced fine
1 tbsp. lemon juice	1 sprig fresh dill, minced
1/2 c. safflower mayonnaise	fine
1/4 c. yogurt	1 sprig fresh summer
2 tbsp. chopped chives	savory, minced fine
2 tbsp. chopped parsley	Freshly ground pepper, no
	salt

Boil potatoes in their jackets until they can be pierced easily with a fork. Cool slightly and dice, with skins on. Combine with other vegetables. Make dressing by dissolving honey in lemon juice and vinegar. Combine mayonnaise and yogurt and pour in honey and vinegar, stirring constantly. Add minced herbs and pepper. Pour dressing over potato mixture while potatoes are still warm. Mix thoroughly and chill in refrigerator for an hour or two. Garnish with ripe tomatoes and chopped chives.

SPROUT SALAD WITH KEFIR CHEESE DRESSING

1 1/2 c. fresh sunflower	1/2 med. green pepper,
sprouts	chopped
1/2 c. radishes, sliced thin	6 scallions, sliced with
	part of green

KEFIR CHEESE DRESSING:

Kefir cheese is a cultured milk product with a lemony tang and a thick smooth texture. If you can't buy it in your area, try substituting tofu and one teaspoon lemon juice.

1 tsp. barley malt
1 tbsp. apple cider vinegar
   or rice wine vinegar
1/4 c. safflower mayonnaise

1/2 c. kefir cheese (or tofu
   and lemon juice)*
1 tbsp. safflower oil
Cayenne pepper, no salt

Dissolve barley malt in apple cider vinegar. Mix mayonnaise and kefir cheese together and gradually pour in honey and vinegar, stirring constantly. Mix in oil and pepper. Pour over salad and toss.
   *To use tofu, purchase firm tofu, drain and mash with fork or cream in blender.

AVOCADO DRESSING

1 sm. sweet onion
1 med. clove garlic
1 very ripe avocado
1/3 c. safflower mayonnaise

1/2 to 1 tsp. chili powder
Dash each cayenne, basil,
   oregano
1 tsp. lemon juice
1 sm. ripe tomato, cut in
   quarters

In food processor equipped with metal blade, process onion and garlic for a few seconds just to get them started. Then add avocado which has been peeled and cut into quarters, mayonnaise and seasonings. Process until smooth. Last, add tomato quarters and process a few seconds until tomato is incorporated. Pour most of the dressing over the salad and mix well. Garnish with remaining dressing and ripe olives. Serve immediately with baked corn chips.

NETHERLANDS SALAD AND DRESSING

1 c. Romaine lettuce, torn in
   bite size pieces
1 c. chopped celery

1/2 c. chopped sweet onion

DRESSING:

1/2 c. safflower mayonnaise
1 tbsp. Dijon-type mustard
1 tsp. barley malt syrup
1 tbsp. apple cider vinegar
1 tbsp. safflower oil
Chopped chives
Cayenne pepper, no salt

Combine lettuce, celery and onion. Mix dressing, pour over salad, toss and serve immediately with whole wheat French bread.

CARROT-LENTIL SALAD

1 c. uncooked dried lentils
2 1/2 c. water
1 bay leaf
1 clove garlic
1 med. onion
4 med. sized raw carrots
6 scallions, chopped with
   part of green
2 tbsp. chopped parsley

Cook lentils in the water with the bay leaf, garlic, and onion until tender, about 30 minutes. Drain and cool. Save the cooking water and freeze it for later use in soups. Wash carrots well, but do not peel. Cut them into quarters, lengthwise, and steam for about 10 minutes until they are just barely tender. Cool and dice. Do not dice the carrots and then steam them, because they will cook too much and will not be the right texture. They should be tender, but with a hint of crispness, not as hard as raw carrots, nor as soft as cooked carrots. In a large non-metal bowl, mix together the lentils, carrots, scallions and parsley.

MEDITTERANEAN CHICKPEA SALAD WITH LEMON-HERB DRESSING

2 c. cooked chickpeas
1 recipe Lemon-Herb
   dressing for marinade
1 med. green pepper, cut in
   strips
1/4 c. chopped sweet onion
2 med. sized ripe tomatoes,
   cut in thin wedges, or
   12 cherry tomatoes,
   halved
2 tbsp. chopped parsley
1 recipe Lemon-Herb
   dressing for salad

Place chickpeas in a non-metal bowl. Pour dressing over them and marinate in the refrigerator for an hour or two. Add rest of ingredients, toss well and serve.
Variation: Add two tablespoons toasted sesame seeds to salad just before serving.

LEMON-HERB DRESSING:

1 fresh squeezed lemon
2 tbsp. olive oil
3 tbsp. distilled water
1/8 tsp. cayenne pepper

1/4 c. brown rice vinegar
2 tsp. fresh basil
1/2 tsp. dry mustard

Mix all ingredients in a blender.

GREEN BEAN SALAD

1 lb. garden-fresh green
  beans
1 med. onion, thinly sliced
1 cucumber, thinly sliced

1 c. yogurt
1 tsp. Gomasio seasoning
2 tbsp. lemon juice

Steam green beans until crisp-tender. Combine with remaining ingredients and chill well before serving. Serves 6 to 8.

TOFU EGG-LESS SALAD

You'll hardly believe it has no eggs!

1 lb. tofu, mashed
1/4 tsp. salt
2 tsp. prepared mustard
1/4 tsp. garlic powder
Cayenne pepper to taste
1 green pepper, minced
1 rib celery, chopped finely

2 to 3 scallions or 1 sm.
  onion, minced,
  optional
1/8 tsp. turmeric, optional
1/2 tsp. soy sauce, optional
1/2 tsp. Gomasio
  seasoning

Mash tofu to a crumbly consistency. Add mustard and seasonings, mix well. Add vegetables and mix again. Serve on lettuce leaves or in sandwiches with lettuce or sprouts. Vary the seasoning to taste and try using other herbs or vegetables like parsley, chives, or grated carrot.

SYRIAN SALAD (TABOULI)

6 lg. tomatoes
1 bunch parsley
1 c. mint leaves
1 1/2 bunch green onions

2 c. cracked wheat
3 lemons, juice
1/4 c. olive oil
Salt and cayenne pepper to taste

Mince the parsley, mint and green onions. Chop the tomatoes. Cover the cracked wheat with boiling water. Let it stand 5 minutes and drain well. Add together with olive oil, lemon juice, salt and cayenne pepper.

RISOTTO SALAD

2 lg. onions, chopped
2 garlic cloves, crushed
2 tbsp. salad oil (unrefined)
4 tomatoes, skinned and diced
1 tomato, slice for garnish
1 1/2 c. brown rice
2 1/2 c. veggie bouillon (unyeasted)

2 carrots, grated
1 box frozen peas
6 oz. sliced mushrooms
3 tbsp. chopped parsley
Salt and cayenne pepper to taste

Boil rice: 1 1/2 cups brown rice to 2 cups water. Saute onions and garlic in oil until clear. Add mushrooms, carrots and peas and 1/2 cup bouillon. Cook 5 minutes or until peas are tender. Add tomato cubes. Remove from fire. Cook rice in remaining bouillon until tender. Add vegetable mixture. Toss with parsley. Garnish top with reserved tomato slices and parsley sprigs. (Also black olives if desired). May be served hot or cold.

SZECHWAN NOODLE SALAD

This wonderful recipe was adapted from an old Szechwan cookbook; originally it is called for cellophane noodles, thin, transparent Chinese noodles made from mung bean flour. My friend Kathy adapted it to use soba, Japanese buckwheat noodles, and this is my favorite version. It's hot, the spiciness can be altered by reducing the cayenne and garlic.

2 (6 oz.) pkg. soba noodles
    or wheat pasta
2 inches gingerroot, grated,
    unpeeled
1 (8 oz.) can sliced water
    chestnuts
1/2 lb. thinly sliced
    mushrooms
1 c.unslated slivered
    almonds or walnuts

1/4 c. sesame oil
10 sm. cloves garlic,
    minced very well
6 minced green onions,
    include greens
2 tsp. Szechwan pepper, or
    cayenne
1/2 c. tamari
1/2 tsp. honey

Cook noodles in boiling water until "al dente", drain and rinse under cold water. Toss with remaining ingredients and serve. Serves 8.

FRESH HERB DRESSING

1 tsp. tamari sauce
2 lemons
1 clove garlic
1 tsp. Gomasio seasoning

1 c. unrefined oil
    (sunflower)
1/4 c. natural rice wine
    vinegar
1 oz. combined dill weed,
    parsley and thyme

Wash, peel and pit the lemons, then liquify at high speed. Peel and halve the garlic and add it to the blender with the Gomasio and oil. Blend until smooth. Wash the parsley well and pat half dry in a towel. Cut parsley into 1 inch pieces and blend with the other ingredients until well chopped. Yield: 1 1/2 cups.

CHICKPEA SPREAD (HOMMUS)

2 tsp. chopped fresh parsley
1 c. chickpeas
3 c. water
1 clove garlic, minced

1/2 c. tahini
2 tbsp. lemon juice
3/4 tsp. sea salt

Soak chickpeas overnight (or boil for 1 minute and soak for 2 hours), add garlic and simmer for 2 to 3 hours until tender. If pressure cooking use 2 1/2 cups water and cook for 1 hour. Combine cooked chickpeas with other ingredients and puree all together in a blender, a food mill, or by mashing with a fork. This Middle Eastern specialty is good on sandwiches with lettuce and/or sprouts, and makes a good dip for crackers when thinned with 1/4 to 1/2 cup water.

PEACH-COCONUT

2 lg. peaches, cut in half
1 sm. peach, peeled

1 tsp. lemon juice
3 tbsp. fresh, grated
   coconut

Remove seeds from large peaches. Brush cut surface with lemon juice. Mash small peach and mix with coconut. Spoon mixture into peach halves. Variation: Omit coconut and use 3 tbsp. sprouted sunflower seeds.

BANANA-PERSIMMON

2 bananas
2 persimmons

3 tbsp. fresh grated
   coconut

Peel and slice bananas lengthwise into halves. Arrange on serving plate, alternating with peeled and sliced persimmons. Sprinkle with coconut.

SUMMER RICE SALAD

2/3 c. cooked rice (brown)
4 tsp. green onion, minced
4 tsp. bell pepper, minced
2 tsp. minced parsley
4 tbsp. sliced jicama or
    turnip, raw
4 tsp. celery, minced
2 sliced radishes

2 tbsp. mayonnaise (to
    taste)
Dash of tamari
1 1/2 tsp. lemon juice
Pinch of cayenne
1 tbsp. light wine
1/2 sm. tomato, seeded
    and cut into strips

Combine and chill.

TOFU-MISO DIP OR FILLING

8 oz. tofu, well drained
2 tbsp. sesame butter

2 tsp. miso (dark or light)
2 tbsp. minced celery,
    optional

Mash the tofu, then add sesame butter and miso. Mix thoroughly and add the celery if desired.

NUTTY OR SEEDY MISO TOPPING

1 c. chopped nuts (or
    sunflower seeds)
4 tbsp. dark miso

3 tbsp. honey
1 tbsp. water

Combine all ingredients in a small skillet and bring to a boil, stirring constantly. Reduce heat and simmer about 2 minutes until mixture thickens. Cool before serving and store refrigerated.
Variations: Omit nuts or use nut butter instead of nuts (reduce amount to 1/3 cup). Add mustard, vinegar, lemon juice, minced garlic or grated onion to taste.

ZUCCHINI AND YOGURT DIP

1 lb. fresh zucchini
1 c. yogurt
2 cloves garlic, crushed
1/2 c. tahini
2 tbsp. lemon juice

1 tsp. salt
1/2 tsp. pepper
2 tbsp. fresh parsley,
    finely chopped

Bake the zucchini in the oven until they become soft, then peel and mash. Add the remaining ingredients (except the parsley) and mix thoroughly. Place on a serving platter and chill. Decorate with the parsley just before serving.

TAHINI-MISO SPREAD

1 tbsp. lemon juice
1/2 c. tahini
1/4 c. water

1 tbsp. miso (or more to
    taste)
2 tbsp. finely chopped
    parsley
2 tbsp. chives

Mix lemon juice with tahini, then slowly add water and mix well until smooth. Add miso and parsley and chives.

FINGERTIP MINI

4 thin circles of carrots
4 slices of broccoli stems,
    peeled
4 slices of cucumbers
4 slices of yellow summer
    squash

4 slices of radishes
1 c. alfalfa sprouts
1/2 c. buckwheat greens

Use toothpicks and alternate the slices to make a colorful appearance. Serve on alfalfa sprouts and buckwheat greens. Perfect for dipping!

CONFETTI RICE SALAD

1/3 c. sunflower seeds
1 1/2 tsp. celery seeds
2/3 c. minced watercress or
    parsley
1/4 c. minced red onion
2 c. cooked brown rice or
    other grain

2 tsp. lemon juice
1/4 c. safflower oil
3 tbsp. cider vinegar
1/8 tsp. dry mustard
1/8 tsp. paprika
Pinch salt

Toast sunflower seeds by stirring in a dry pan on medium heat for a few minutes until they start to give off a nice fragrance. Add celery seeds and stir a bit until their fragrance just starts to come out. Remove from pan at once. Mix vegetables, seeds, rice, and lemon juice in a good sized salad bowl. Mix oil, vinegar, and seasonings well to make dressing. Mix dressing with vegetable-rice mixture and let sit in refrigerator to marinate for 1/2 hour, before serving.

WHOLE MEAL SALAD WITH MISO SAUCE

3 c. cooked long grain brown rice
1/2 c. chopped green onions
1/4 c. chopped parsley
3/8 tsp. dry mustard
2 tbsp. minced garlic

1/4 c. vinegar
1/8 c. lemon juice
1/4 tsp. salt
Dash of cayenne pepper
1/4 c. each olive oil and safflower oil

Combine all ingredients and let marinate at room temperature for 1 hour. Then serve with the following salad and miso sauce.

SALAD:

1 c. mixed sprouts
1/2 green pepper, chopped
1/4 c. sliced Jerusalem artichoke
1 stalk celery, chopped
2 tomatoes, quartered

1 c. cooked potatoes, cold, cubed
1 lg. beet, steamed and shredded
1 c. shredded green cabbage

Combine in layers all ingredients, placing the marinated rice mixture on the bottom. Serve with:

MISO SAUCE:

1 1/2 tbsp. light miso
3/4 c. safflower oil
1/4 c. each: tamari, vinegar and water

1 tsp. grated ginger
3 tbsp. honey

Combine in blender and serve over salad. This dressing keeps for 2 months in the refrigerator. This whole meal salad serves 6.

BROWN RICE SALAD

2 c. cooked long grain brown
   rice
1 c. shredded carrots
4 oz. red bell peppers
1/2 c. minced scallions

1 c. fresh peas, or cooked
   beans
1 tbsp. olive or sesame oil
1 avocado, optional
Bed of lettuce

    Cook rice day before and chill. For directions to cook rice, refer to recipe and Brown Rice Casserole. Next day, shred carrots, cut peppers and avocados into cubes and add to rice.
    Add fresh peas and oil. Serve on a bed of lettuce. May be served with Marscell's peanut butter dressing. Makes 2 ample servings.

Exciting Entrees

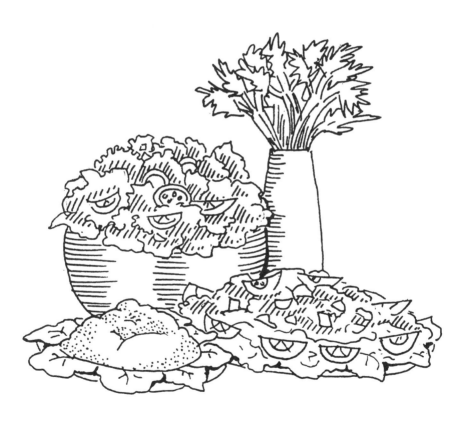

FELAFEL SANDWICHES

1 c. dried garbanzo beans
2 cloves garlic, minced
2 tbsp. fresh parsley,
   minced
1/4 tsp. cumin
1 tbsp. sesame tahini

Dash cayenne
2 tbsp. lemon juice
1/2 tsp. salt
Fine dry whole wheat
   bread crumbs, about
   1/2 c.

Soak the garbanzo beans overnight. Sprout 3 or 4 days until sprouts are about 1/2 inch long. In a food processor or blender, grind together the beans, garlic, parsley, cumin, tahini, cayenne, lemon juice and salt. Form balls about 1 inch in diameter. Roll them in the bread crumbs. Place on a cookie sheet and bake at 350 degrees for 25 minutes, turning twice.

DRESSING:

1 to 3 cloves garlic, finely
   minced
4 tbsp. lemon juice

3 tbsp. tahini (or enough
   to make a thick
   dressing)
Pinch each cayenne and
   cumin

Mix all ingredients together thoroughly.

SANDWICHES:

1 sm. cucumber, finely
   chopped
1 med. tomato, peeled,
   seeded and chopped
4 scallions, minced

2 oz. alfalfa or mixed
   sprouts
Plain yogurt (optional)
Whole wheat pita bread

Mix the dressing with the cucumber, tomato, scallions and alfalfa sprouts. Cut each pita in half. Place a spoonful of the vegetables in the pocket. Top with hot felafels. Lavish with yogurt or tahini-miso dressing.

HOMMUS

1/4 c. olive oil
1 c. garbanzos
3 c. water
3 cloves garlic, minced

1/2 c. sesame tahini
1/4 c. lemon juice
3/4 tsp. sea salt

Soak garbanzos overnight, add garlic and simmer for 2 to 3 hours until tender. If pressure cooking use 2 1/2 cups water and cook for 1 hour. Combine cooked garbanzos with other ingredients and puree all together; in a blender or food processor. Can be thinned with water to make a dip.

SPINACH FETTUCINE WITH WHITE MUSHROOM SAUCE

2 c. fresh soymilk
16 med. size mushrooms
3 to 5 cloves garlic, halved
1 1/2 tbsp. rice or whole wheat flour (rice flour gives a lighter texture)

1/4 tsp. sea salt
1 lb. cooked spinach fettucine pasta
A pinch of nutmeg
Italian pepper, crushed to taste

Combine soymilk, all the mushrooms and garlic in a heavy bottom saucepan. Place over moderate heat and cook for 7 minutes, never allowing the soy milk to boil. Stir often.
Puree mixture along with flour in a blender or food processor. Return mixture to saucepan and cook over low heat, stirring often until sauce is slightly thickened, about 7 minutes. Just before done add a pinch of nutmeg and a pinch of crushed Italian red pepper. Serve over cooked spinach fettucine pasta and Enjoy!

DAIRYLESS PASTA AL PESTO

1/2 c. spinach leaves, washed and dried
1/2 c. fresh parsley
2 tbsp. unrefined bottled olive oil
2 cloves fresh garlic, minced
1 tbsp. light white miso

1/4 c. walnuts or pine nuts
1 tbsp. fresh basil
1 lb. natural jerusalem artichoke or thin spinach pasta, boiled until tender and drained

In a blender or food processor, mix together the garlic, nuts, and olive oil. Add white miso and blend 30 seconds. Add basil spinach, parsley; blend briefly until "paste-like" consistency. Finally, just toss with hot pasta. NOTE: For a change of pace try buckwheat soba or rice noodles.

CHUNKY EGGPLANT AND ROSEMARY SAUCE

1 lg. eggplant, diced with skin on
2 med. onions, chopped coarsely
3 cloves garlic, chopped
4 c. fresh chopped tomatoes
2 tbsp. rosemary
2 stalks celery, chopped
1 tsp. cayenne to pepper, or
1/2 c. fresh chopped parsley
2 to 3 tbsp. olive oil
1 c. stock (vegetable)

Chop onions, garlic and celery. Heat oil in a large pot and saute vegetables for 5 minutes until golden. Sprinkle with rosemary.

Dice eggplant and add to pot. Stir briefly, then add tomatoes with their juices (make sure they are not the pink plastic winter variety - they do not have enough flavor or juice). Allow the sauce to come to a boil, then add stock. Bring to the boil again and reduce to a simmer, uncovered.

Put on water for pasta. Add cayenne pepper and half the parsley and continue to simmer sauce uncovered.

When the water has boiled, add pasta, stirring until the strands have separated and the water is boiling madly. If the pasta is fresh, boil only two to three minutes, until al dente, still slightly firm, but not soft; if dried, it may need to boil up to seven minutes. Test it occasionally. Drain and transfer pasta to a warm bowl, pour the eggplant sauce on top and toss. Serve immediately garnished with parsley and cayenne pepper.

RED SNAPPER EN PAPILLOTE

2 lbs. red snapper fillets, or other fresh fillets
1 med. green pepper, sliced into rings
1 med. onion, sliced into rings
1/4 c. melted butter or soy margarine
2 tbsp. lemon juice
1 tsp. tamari
1 tsp. paprika
1 slice fresh ginger, grated

Brush fillets with half the melted butter and sprinkle with seasonings. Saute onion, green pepper and ginger in rest of butter or margarine in large skillet for 5 minutes. Place fillets on top of vegetables, cover and cook for 10 to 15 minutes, until fish flakes with a fork.

MUSHROOM PATE'

1/2 lg. onion, chopped
2 scallions, chopped
4 cloves garlic, minced
1 1/2 c. mushrooms, minced
2 tbsp. sherry
1 tbsp. olive oil
2 stalks celery, minced

1/2 c. walnuts
1/2 c. bread crumbs, whole grain
1 pinch rosemary
1/2 tsp. thyme
1 tbsp. tamari sauce
1/2 tsp. basil, fresh, of course

Heat oil in skillet and add onion. Saute, stirring, until limp but not browned. Add mushrooms, garlic and sherry. Saute one - two minutes until mushrooms begin to juice. Stir in rosemary, thyme, tamari, salt and basil. Put remaining ingredients into food processor and combine until minced. Add mushroom mixture and blend. Put mixture into bowl and refrigerate two hours. Spread on bread and crackers or hollow out a loaf of French bread and stuff.

STUFFED ARTICHOKES

Wash and cut tops off, removing about 1/2 inch. Put in pot of boiling water for 5 minutes, remove and fill each leaf with the following mixture:

Finely grated cornbread crumbs or 1/4 c. cornmeal
1 tbsp. fresh parsley
1 tsp. fresh basil

1/2 tsp. powdered garlic
1/4 cayenne pepper
1 tsp. Gomasio seasoning

Fill each leaf with a tablespoon of mixture. Put artichokes back in pot in 1 inch of water, pour a little cold pressed safflower oil over each artichoke. Simmer until leaf comes off easily, 15 to 20 minutes, low medium heat. Serves 2.

STIR FRIED VEGGIES FU YUNG

Use all fresh ingredients.

1 slice fresh ginger
1 thinly sliced yellow
  squash
1 thinly sliced green pepper
1 thinly sliced Jersulem
  artichoke (sun chokes)
1 thinly sliced green onion
  (scallion)
1/2 c. sliced mushrooms

1 thinly sliced carrot
1 thinly sliced stalk of
  celery
4 spears chopped broccoli
1/2 c. mung sprouts
3 tbsp. tamari
1/2 c. safflower oil, cold
  pressed
2 beaten eggs, add last
  (optional)
3 cloves minced garlic

Heat wok for 5 minutes with safflower oil in it. Add all ingredients, except sprouts and eggs. Season with 2 tsp. Gomasio seasoning. Keep turning veggies for 8 minutes over medium low heat. Add sprouts, stir for 1 minute. Pour eggs over veggies. Lower heat. Simmer until egg is cooked. Serve at once.

SUSHI PLATTERS

1 strip kombu (seaweed)
1/4 c. rice vinegar (optional)
2 tbsp. barley-malt syrup

3 c. cooked brown rice
Nori seaweed

For the filling choose from: sliced, toasted, scallions; cooked spinach; sliced lengthwise carrots; powdered or pressed horseradish; sliced avocado, pickled sliced ginger, and umaboshi plum paste.

Heat the vinegar, barley-malt syrup, and kombu until boiling. Lower heat and simmer for 5 minutes. Remove kombu and pour over rice; mix well.

Spread rice on sheets of toasted nori seaweed. Place filling of your choice in center. Roll into tight roll and let sit to seal. Cut carefully into circles.

ASPARAGUS POLONAISE

2 tbsp. unrefined safflower
  seed oil
1/4 c. chopped Fu

2 lbs. asparagus, cooked
Chopped parsley, for
  garnish

In small skillet, heat the oil and add the bread crumbs. Saute until lightly browned. Sprinkle the crumbs over the hot, freshly cooked asparagus spears. Sprinkle the minced parsley over all. Yield: 4 servings.

BOILED ASPARAGUS

Remove the tough ends by snapping them off. Using a vegetable peeler, peel the stalks. Plunge into boiling salted water, just to cover. Cook until just tender, about 8 to 10 minutes for the medium stalks.

Prepared this way, asparagus may be served with melted butter and lemon or unrefined safflower seed oil and unfiltered apple cider vinegar.

STIR FRY LENTILS (SPROUTED)

Sprout 1/4 cup lentils about 5 days. Place in sun last day to green.

1 c. chopped green pepper
1 c. sliced celery
1/2 c. green onion, sliced fine
1 c. sliced mushrooms

1/4 c. sliced sunchokes, optional
1/2 c. raw broccoli buds (optional)
1/4 c. raw cashews, optional

Stir fry or saute everything except lentils in hot pan for about 3 minutes. Throw in rinsed and drained lentils and add two scant teaspoons tamari. Cook one more minute. Serve immediately with brown rice. Serves about 6 people.

KASHA PILAF

1 tbsp. olive oil
1 onion, minced
1 stalk celery, minced
1 green pepper, minced

2 cloves garlic, minced
1 c. whole kasha
4 c. stock
4 tbsp. tamari

Heat the oil in a large, heavy pot and saute the onion, celery, pepper and garlic until the onion is limp. Stir in the kasha until coated with oil. Add the stock and tamari. Bring to a boil, cover and simmer over low heat 20 minutes.

EGGPLANT AUBERGINE CONTINENTAL

Bake whole eggplant, poke with a fork a couple of times, and while it cooks:
1. Chop 1 onion, 1 seeded green pepper, and 1 tomato into very fine pieces. 2. Add 1 thinly sliced zucchini and 1 clove of minced garlic. 3. Heat 4 tbsp. of safflower oil in a large skillet and saute the mixture until ingredients are limp and tender (do not overcook). 4. Peel eggplant, chop it very fine and add to skillet. 5. Add 3 tbsp. of red wine (optional), 1/2 tbsp. oregano, 1/2 tsp. Gomasio seasoning, 1/4 tsp. cayenne pepper.

Mix all together and stir in 2 tbsp. brown rice miso, then simmer for 40 minutes. Serve hot or cold as a dip.

PASTA E FAGIOLI

3/4 c. garbanzo beans
3/4 c. navy beans
1 1/2 qts. water
1 lg. onion, chopped
2 carrots, thinly sliced
2 stalks celery, chopped
1 lg. ripe tomato, chopped
2 bay leaves
4 cloves fresh minced garlic

2 tbsp. miso
1 tsp. dried thyme
Salt, to taste
Virgin olive oil, optional
Cayenne pepper, to taste
8 oz. fettucine noodles,
    small elbows or shell
    pasta (whole wheat,
    artichoke, or
    buckwheat)

Combine beans and wash well. Place in a large pot and cover with cold water. Allow beans to soak 6 hours or overnight.

Drain and rinse again; place in a pot with 1 1/2 quarts of water. Bring to a boil, cover pot, reduce heat and cook at a simmer until beans are almost done, about two hours. Add more water to keep beans covered as they cook, if necessary.

Add onion, carrots, celery, tomato, bay leaves, thyme, garlic and miso and cook 30 minutes longer. Add salt to taste.

Cook pasta separately in lightly salted water; drain and combine with beans and vegetables. Garnish each serving with a sprinkling of olive oil, if desired, and cayenne pepper and parsley.

CREOLE

1 lb. fresh fish fillets, cut in 1 inch chunks
1/4 c. vegetable oil
1/4 c. whole wheat flour
1 c. hot water
1/2 lb. fresh tomatoes
1/2 c. chopped green onions and tops
1/2 c. chopped parsley
1/4 c. chopped green pepper
4 cloves garlic, minced
2 whole bay leaves
1 1/2 tsp. salt
1/2 tsp. thyme
Dash cayenne pepper
1 lemon slice
Cooked brown rice

Prepare roux by heating oil in large skillet and blending in flour over medium heat. Stir constantly until brown, being careful not to scorch. Add water gradually and cook until thick and smooth. Add remaining ingredients except rice. Cover and simmer for 15 minutes. Remove bay leaves and serve over hot rice.

RED SNAPPER VERA CRUZ

1 to 3 lbs. red snapper, or similar white fish, filleted
3 tbsp. fresh lime juice
6 tbsp. olive oil
1 med. onion, chopped
2 cloves garlic, minced
2 lbs. skinned chopped tomatoes
1 bay leaf
1/2 tsp. oregano
1/2 c. green olives, sliced (natural style)
Salt to taste

To prepare fish, prick with a fork and cover with lime juice. Let fish sit for about 2 hours. Sprinkle with 2 tbsp. of olive oil. Cover with the following tomato sauce:

Heat 4 tbsp. of olive oil. Add the chopped onion and minced garlic. Saute until soft. Add 2 lbs. of chopped tomatoes and bay leaf, oregano, green olives and salt to taste. Cook the sauce until some of the juices have evaporated.

Pour the tomato sauce over the fish and bake at 350 degrees for 10 to 12 minutes or until the fish flakes with a fork. Avoid over cooking or the fish will become tough and dry.

TEMPEH TURKEY WITH SAVORY GRAVY

2 lbs. tempeh
1 c. oil, for frying

SAVORY STOCK:

3 c. water or stock
1 to 2 tbsp. miso
1 tbsp. prepared mustard
1/2 sage leaf

1/4 tsp. rosemary
1/2 tsp. thyme
2 to 3 tbsp. kuzu, dissolved
in 1/4 c. water

Cut tempeh into 2 inch triangles. Slice each triangle in half; one pound will yield 24 thin, bite size triangles. Heat oil in heavy pan, fry tempeh until golden brown. Drain in paper towel. Place fried tempeh in a saucepan. Mix savory stock together and pour over tempeh. Bring broth to a boil, lower flame, simmer at least 1/2 to 1 hour. Long, slow simmering results in tender and delicious tempeh.

After tempeh is tender, dissolve kuzu in water. Stir into broth with tempeh. Continue to stir until sauce thickens. Turn off flame. Cover. Reheat slowly when ready to serve. Adjust seasonings. Serve over wild rice stuffing.

TOFU BURRITOS

2 c. tofu, squeezed and
shredded
2 c. hot salsa
8 whole wheat flour
tortillas (warmed by
wrapping in a tea towel
and placing in
steamer or oven)

1 c. radish sprouts
1/2 c. chopped tomatoes
2 c. black beans, cooked
1 c. seitan

Place the mashed tofu in a bowl with 1 cup of the salsa. Let this mixture marinate at room temperature for 30 minutes. Meanwhile, prepare the other ingredients and heat the beans in a saucepan. Mince the seitan to have consistency of chopped meat. To assemble the burritos, place a large spoonful of the tofu-salsa mixture in the lower corner of the tortilla. Layer beans, then seitan, sprouts, tomato and more salsa over the tofu. Roll the burrito away from you, folding in the two sides and tucking the top edge under as you roll. Bake on a non stick surface for 10 to 15 minutes, then serve. Add more salsa if desired, hot stuff!

STIR FRY TOFU WITH MISO AND SPAGHETTI

Whole wheat pasta tends to be heavy; I prefer the soy/-sesame noodles, rice noodles or buckwheat sorba. Immerse:

2/3 lb. spaghetti in   **1 tsp. oil has been added**
2 qts. boiling, salted water
to which

Keep at a rolling boil until spaghetti is done. Drain. While spaghetti boils, saute:

1/2 lb. cubed tofu in   **1/2 tsp. oil**

As the water in the tofu evaporates, douse it liberally with tamari. As the tamari evaporates, it leaves a thin crust on tofu cubes; stir frequently to prevent burning. When tofu and pasta are done, combine them in the skillet and add:

1 tbsp. olive oil   **2 tsp. fresh basil**
1 to 2 tbsp. dark miso   **Sea salt to taste**
creamed in
1/4 c. water

Mix well and serve with a crisp green salad.

SPICY FRIED TOFU

A showcase for tofu's natural affinity for spices and seasonings, good in sandwiches or tacos with tomato and shredded lettuce.

1 tbsp. miso   **1/2 tsp. each turmeric and**
Safflower oil for frying   **thyme**
2 lb. tofu   **1/2 to 3/4 tsp. curry**
1/4 tsp. basil   **2 cloves garlic pressed**
1 tsp. dill weed   **2 tbsp. shoyu**
                                    2 tsp. Gomasio seasoning

First press tofu by cutting into 1/2 inch slices and firmly patting out the excess water with an absorbent towel. Cut into small cubes. Heat 3 tbsp. oil in a skillet or wok on high heat. Add tofu and saute for 5 minutes, turning with a spatula. If more water comes out while sauteeing. Tip pan and remove it with a spoon. Reduce heat to medium, add turmeric and stir until tofu is yellow all over. Add dill weed, basil, thyme, curry and Gomasio seasoning, stirring well between each. Add the garlic and two more tbsp. oil to prevent the tofu from sticking. Increase heat and add shoyu, stirring constantly. Good hot or cold, serves four to eight.

SCRAMBLED TOFU

3 tbsp. sesame seed oil
1 tbsp. tamari, optional
1/2 c. sauteed scallions

1/2 tsp. sea salt
2 c. crumbled tofu
1/2 tsp. Gomasio
    seasoning

Add to skillet and mix until seasonings are evenly distributed. Heat and serve like scrambled eggs.

VEGETARIAN TOFU CHILI

2 c. cooked and drained
    kidney beans
1 c. frozen tofu, thawed,
    squeezed dry and
    mashed
2 lbs. mushrooms, sliced
3 sm. onions, chopped
    coarsely
1/2 c. mild chilies, minced
1/2 c. tamari
1/2 c. red wine, optional

4 lg. cloves minced garlic
1 tbsp. sesame oil
1 c. each, minced: green
    pepper, celery, carrot
1 tsp. each: cumin and
    basil
1 tsp. chili powder, to taste

Mix together the tofu, wine, tamari, cumin, basil and chili powder; let marinade at room temperature for 1 hour. Meanwhile, heat the oil in a large soup pot and saute the onion until limp but not browned. Add the carrot, celery and green pepper. Saute 2 minutes. Add mushrooms and garlic, and saute until mushrooms begin to exude moisture, about 5 minutes at fairly high heat. Add all remaining ingredients, including tofu marinade, and bring to a boil. Lower heat and simmer for 1 hour or until chili is thick and fragrant and the seasonings are well blended. Season to taste and serve with hot cornbread.

GINGERY MISO BROTH WITH CARROT FLOWERS

2 qts. stock or water
2 sm. strips kombu (sea
    vegetable)
3 to 4 shiitake mushrooms
2 tsp. fresh ginger
1/4 c. miso (shiro or kome)

1/2 c. water
2/3 carrots for flowers
3 scallions, sliced thin for
    garnish

Rinse komu and shiitake mushrooms, place in stock or water. Add ginger. Bring to a boil, lower flame, simmer for 1/2 hour. Remove kombu and shiitake. Slice kombu into long 1 inch strips, then slice across strips thinly. Cut mushroom stems off caps. Slice mushroom caps thinly. Return kombu and shiitake to stock. Simmer gently. Cut carrot flowers, add to stock 10 minutes before serving, so the carrots will cook slightly. Five minutes before serving, add miso dissolved in 1/2 cup water.

STUFFED MUSHROOM CAPS WITH TOFU

12 lg. mushrooms (caps and stems separated)
3 tbsp. soy oil or safflower oil margarine
1 sm. onion, minced or grated
1/2 c. Fu crumbs
1/2 c. frozen tofu, thawed, squeezed dry and mashed
1/4 c. chopped almonds or cashews
2 tbsp. sherry or white wine
Pinch of sea salt and cayenne pepper
Pinch of marjoram
1 tbsp. tamari sauce

Mince the mushroom stems in a processor or by hand. Mix together with the Fu crumbs and tofu. Add the sherry or wine, seasonings and tamari and let marinate 15 minutes. Place the mushrooms caps face down on an ungreased baking sheet. Preheat broiler; lightly broil mushroom caps until dry and wrinkled looking. Turn over and broil 1/2 minute face up. Let cool.

Heat margarine in saucepan and saute onion until soft but not browned. Add tofu marinated mixture and nuts, and saute 2 minutes. Mound this mixture into the mushroom caps, filling as high as possible. Garnish with gomasio seasoning and broil until light brown. Serve warm.

CARROT-ALMOND PATE

1 1/2 c. almonds
2 c. grated carrots, chopped fine
2 tbsp. tamari
1 to 1 1/2 c. water
3 tbsp. eggless soy mayonnaise

Blend almonds into a nut meal (raw and roasted will give different tastes). Blend in remaining ingredients until smooth, adding water to desired thickness. Let sit in refrigerator about 30 minutes before serving. Can be used as a dip for, or served on top of, crackers and raw vegetable slices as a canape.

CANDIED YAMS

2 lbs. yams
1 tsp. sesame oil
1 to 2 tsp. tamari
1/2 c. apple juice or water

GLAZE:

2 to 3 tbsp. barley malt, dissolved in 1/4 cup water or orange juice 1 tsp. sesame oil. Peel yams. Slice into 1/4 to 1/2 inch rounds. Line baking/serving dish neatly with yams. Mix oil, tamari and liquid together; pour over yams. Cover and bake at 375 degrees for 45 to 60 minutes.

Mix barley malt, water and oil together, brush or pour over cooked yams, to give a glazed look. Cover, keep warm.

KALE

Wash one bunch of kale greens well. If the leaves are large, slice down the middle along the stalk; if small, leave whole. Drop in boiling water and cook uncovered for 5 to 10 minutes, depending on how you like them. Drain and serve.

WATERCRESS

Wash one bunch very well. Boil 3 cups water in a skillet. Drop watercress in boiling water for no more than 1 minute; then remove, chop and place in small bowl. Add the following sauce:

Mix 3 tbsp. almond butter and 3 tbsp. light miso with distilled water to desired consistency. Should make approximately 1/2 to 3/4 cup.

CRANBERRY KANTEN

1 qt. apple juice
1/2 c. agar flakes, or one bar
   agar
1 tbsp. kuzu
2 apples, diced
2 c. cranberries
1/2 c. roasted, chopped
   walnuts
1 orange peel, grated and
   juiced
Pinch of salt
1/4 tsp. cinnamon,
   optional
1/4 c. barley malt is
   optional for extra
   sweetness

"Kanten" is a name given to dishes thickened with agar-agar. To make this one, pour juice in a saucepan. Add agar and stir; bring to a low boil, then simmer for 20 minutes until agar is completely dissolved. While mixture is cooking, dice apple, grate orange, roast and chop walnuts, wash cranberries.

When kanten has cooked for 20 minutes, dissolve kuzu in 1/4 cup water; stir kuzu into kanten, continue to stir until the kuzu cooks and becomes clear. Now add the remaining ingredients. Simmer 2 to 3 minutes until the cranberries "pop".

Pour into a low, shallow serving dish. Allow to cool to room temperature, then place in the refrigerator.

Serve with the meal or as a dessert. This dish is best if made the day before.

MUSHROOM RISSOULES

Individual pyramid-shaped mushroom roasts to serve with cashew or brown gravy. A good choice for those who like to plan ahead, as the mixture should be chilled before shaping.

3 tbsp. oil Canola
1/2 lb. mushrooms, chopped (about 3 c.)
1/2 c. chopped scallions
2 stalks celery, minced
2 tsp. Gomasio seasoning
1/2 c. soy milk
2 tbsp. soy flour

2 eggs, lightly beaten
1 tsp. salt or Tamari
1 c. cornmeal
1/2 c. combined walnuts and sunflower seeds, ground

Heat 2 tablespoons oil in a skillet or small saucepan and saute mushrooms, onion, celery and Gomasio seasoning for 10 minutes. Gradually stir milk into soy flour and stir this mixture into mushrooms. Cook, stirring, for 3 to 5 minutes until thickened. Remove from heat and cool slightly.

Add eggs, salt, cornmeal and nutmeal. Chill for several hours for easier shaping. preheat oven to 375 degrees. Form mixture into 6 to 8 mounds. Dredge with wheat germ. Place on an oiled baking sheet and drizzle with remaining tablespoon oil. Bake for 30 minutes.

Prepare a gravy while rissoles bake and spoon on top to serve. Serves 4. Variation: For an egg free version, increase milk to 1 cup and soy flour to 1/4 cup.

CHICKPEAS ON THE HALF SHELL

2 acorn squash
1 tbsp. safflower oil
    margarine
1 clove garlic, cut in half
3 slices of Fu, toasted, diced
    into small cubes
1 tbsp. oil - Sesame
1 med. onion, chopped

1/2 c. chopped green
    pepper
1/4 tsp. cayenne
1/4 tsp. cumin
2 tbsp. minced fresh
    parsley
1 1/2 c. cooked chickpeas,
    drained

Preheat oven to 365 degrees. Cut squash in half lengthwise through stem. Scoop out seeds and set in a baking dish, cavity up. Surround with 1/2 inch hot water, cover pan and bake for about 30 minutes until just tender.

While squash bakes, melt butter in a skillet, add garlic and cook for 1 minute. Add Fu cubes and cook, stirring several times, until browned. Transfer Fu to a plate.

Add oil to the skillet and saute onion and green pepper for 3 to 5 minutes until tender. Add cumin and mix well, heating for about 30 seconds longer. Remove from heat and add parsley and chickpeas.

Drain any liquid that has accumulated in the squash. Fill hollow with bean mixture. Cover with croutons, pressing them gently into the surface so they hold.

Return pan, uncovered, to the oven and bake for about 15 minutes, or until filling is hot and squash is tender. Sprinkle with cayenne pepper.

NOTE: Partial baking and stuffing can be done in advance for convenience, and the squash can be refrigerated if it is being held for more than an hour. For best flavor and a moist squash, reserve final baking until just before serving. Be sure to mix the squash meat with the filling as you eat from the shell.

WILD RICE STUFFING

1/2 c. blanched almonds
1/2 c. wild rice, boiled in 2
    c. water
2 c. brown rice, boiled in 4 c.
    water

Pinch of salt
2 to 3 scallions, sliced fine
    for garnish
3 cloves garlic

The wild rice can be boiled separately in 2 cups water for 30 to 40 minutes, then mixed together with brown rice that has been boiled or pressure cooked for 50 to 60 minutes. Or if preferred, boil them together. However, the wild rice will be fluffier if cooked separately.

Saute almonds, scallions and garlic in 3 tbsp. sesame seed oil, then add to rice after rice is cooked and strained.

VEGETABLE DIPPERS

2 to 3 carrots, cut in sticks
or curled with a
vegetable peeler
4 to 5 stalks celery, cut in
sticks
1 bunch radishes, cut in
flowers
2 cucumbers, cut diagonally

1 sm. bunch scallions, cut
in 3 inch pieces
1 sm. jar dill pickles
1 pt. olives, optional

Assemble vegetables on a platter, surrounding a small dish of tofu dip.

CABBAGE AU NATUREL

1/2 cabbage, coarsely sliced
1/4 c. apple cider vinegar
1/2 c. water
1/4 c. safflower oil
2 cloves pressed garlic

1 sliced onion
1/4 tsp. thyme
1/2 tsp. nutmeg
1 1/2 tsp. fresh dill weed

Saute onion in oil with garlic, add cabbage and rest of ingredients. Cook 45 minutes over low medium flame or bake in oven at 400 degrees for 45 minutes.

SPINACH MUSHROOM QUICHE

1/2 c. green scallions,
minced
3 eggs
1 1/2 c. soy milk
2 1/2 c. mashed tofu
1 c. cooked spinach
1/2 c. mushrooms
1/4 c. black olives
1/4 c. chives

1/2 tsp. Gomasio
seasoning
1/4 tsp. cumin
1/2 tsp. garlic powder
3 tbsp. light miso (mix in
1/4 c. water)
Whole wheat crust,
optional

You can make this with or without a crust. Saute mushrooms and olives in cold pressed safflower oil margarine. Combine tofu and soymilk. Mix ingredients in bowl and pour into crust or directly into well greased pie pan or 10 inch glass baking dish.

Bake crust at 450 degrees for 8 minutes, then put in filling. Top with a sprinkle of paprika and minced scallions. Bake at 325 degrees for 40 minutes. Serve hot or at room temperature. You may substitute the eggs for and additional 1 1/2 cups of mashed Tofu.

ROASTED SUNFLOWER AND PUMPKIN SEEDS

1 c. sunflower seeds	2 tsp. tamari
1 c. pumpkin seeds	

On separate baking dishes, spread seeds out evenly. Bake in 325 degree oven. Stir occasionally to roast evenly. Check after 10 minutes. When seeds are golden, sprinkle with tamari and stir to coat evenly. Allow to cool. Store in a jar.

Seeds or nuts can be roasted three to four days ahead of party. Variation: Almonds, pecans or filberts can be tamari-roasted too.

CREAMY PEARL ONIONS

1 to 2 lbs. pearl onions	1/4 tsp. salt or tamari to
2 to 3 tbsp. Kuzu or	taste
arrowroot	2 to 3 tbsp. tahini,
	optional

To peel onions, drop in pot of boiling water for 60 seconds. Drain onions, discard liquid. Onions should slip out of skins easily. Place peeled onions in heavy saucepan with water to cover. Bring to a boil and simmer 20 to 30 minutes until onions are tender.

Dissolve kuzu or arrowroot in 1/4 cup water. Slowly stir in onions. Continue stirring over medium heat until thickened. Lower heat and simmer for five minutes. Add tahini, dissolved in a blender with a little water, if desired. Cover, keep warm until served.

TEMPEH-OLIVE SPREAD

1 pkg. tempeh, cut into
   cubes
1 tbsp. safflower or other
   light oil
2 tbsp. tamari or soy sauce
1/4 c. mayonnaise
   (safflower, eggless)
1 tbsp. minced scallion

1/4 c. minced celery
A handful of chopped ripe
   black olives
A pinch of dill
Cayenne pepper

Steam the tempeh cubes for 20 minutes. Heat the oil in a skillet and lightly saute the tempeh for two to three minutes. Take pan off heat and sprinkle in tamari and toss with the tempeh. Mash tempeh with a fork and mix with other ingredients. Serve with crackers or on whole wheat bread for a sandwich spread.

SZECHWAN VEGETABLES WITH SPICY ALMOND SAUCE

1/2 c. grated or sliced
   carrots
1 lb. tofu, cut into small
   chunks
2 green onions, cut into
   slivers
2 tbsp. grated fresh ginger
   (peeled)

2 tbsp. white wine or
   sherry, optional
1/2 tsp. honey
2 tbsp. water
1 tbsp. safflower oil

Heat the oil in wok or skillet until sizzling hot (drop a small piece of onion in to test). Stir in ginger and carrots. Stir fry over medium high heat until crisp tender. Add wine, water and tofu. Cover and let steam three minutes. Add honey and green onion slivers. Turn off heat. Let sit one minute, covered. Stir in the following almond sauce. Serves 4.

ALMOND SAUCE:

2 tbsp. almond butter
3/4 tsp. cayenne
2 1/2 tbsp. sesame oil
1 tbsp. barley-malt
   sweetener

2 tbsp. tamari
2 tsp. rice vinegar
1 tbsp. green onion
   scallion
1 1/2 tbsp. coriander

Mix together the almond butter, cayenne and oil in a small bowl. When smooth, add remaining ingredients. Combine well and pour over stir fried vegetables. Toss and serve.

BIELER'S BROTH

CELERY, PARSLEY, ZUCCHINI, STRING BEANS
Steam veggies then place in blender with pure water. You may puree or finely chop mixture. You may add fresh garlic and a little Quik-Sip (Bernard Jensen's) to taste. Heat, do not boil.

Eat or drink this broth two to three times daily. This broth will allow you to detoxify while balancing your electrolytes.

CORIANDER AND GARLIC CRISP TEMPEH

We and generations of Indonesian cooks have experimented with many natural seasonints to use with tempeh. All agree that coriander and garlic are the most delicious.

1/2 tsp. ground coriander	6 oz. (170 gm) tempeh, cut
1 clove of garlic, crushed	into slices about 1 by 2
1/2 c. of water	by 1/8 inch thick
2 tsp. salt	Oil for sauteeing

Combine the first four ingredients in a bowl, mixing well. Dip in tempeh slices quickly, then drain briefly on absorbent (paper) toweling or on a rack. Pat surface lightly to absorb excess moisture. Heat the oil to 350 degrees (175 degrees) in a wok or skillet. Slide in tempeh and deep or shallow fry for 3 to 4 minutes, or until crisp and golden brown. Drain briefly on fresh paper toweling and serve immediately either as is (as an hors d'oeuvre or side dish), as an accompaniment for (brown) rice, or as an ingredient in other tempeh recipes.

VARIATIONS:

Seasoned Crisp Tempeh: Prepare as above but omit the coriander and garlic.

Savory Deep-Fried Tempeh: Without dipping tempeh slices in any seasoning solution, deep fry them as described above. Drain briefly, then serve seasoned with a sprinkling of shoyu (natural soy sauce), salt, ketchup, Teriyaki sauce, or Worcestershire sauce.

Crisp Tempeh Chips: After dipping tempeh slices in coriander-and-garlic seasoning solution, dust each slice with whole wheat flour or brown rice flour before frying.

TEMPEH "MOCK CHICKEN" SALAD

6 oz. tempeh, steamed for 20 minutes, allow to cool, and cut into 3/8 inch cubes
4 to 5 tbsp. mayonnaise (tofu, soy milk, or egg)
1 stalk celery, chopped fine
2 tbsp. minced dill pickles

2 tbsp. minced onion
2 tbsp. minced parsley
1 tsp. prepared mustard
1 tsp. shoyu (natural soy sauce)
Dash of garlic powder

Combine all ingredients, mixing lightly but well. Serve as a sandwich filling or mounded on a bed of lettuce.

TEMPEH SHISH KEBAB

Cut tempeh into eight pieces, each 1 by 1 by 3/8 inch thick, then make these into Coriander and Garlic Crisp Tempeh (or any of its variations, described above). If desired, brush finished tempeh lightly with Teriyaki Sauce, then skewer alternately with the following ingredients: pineapple chunks, tomato wedges, small mushrooms, and green pepper chunks.

This recipe can also be prepared without frying: simply marinate the tempeh pieces for 30 minutes in Teriyaki Sauce, then skewer with vegetables and grill over a barbecue or under an oven broiler.

GARBANZO BEAN CASSEROLE

8 oz. cooked garbanzo beans
1/2 c. green onions
1 lb. tomatoes
6 oz. carrots or celery

2 oz. bell peppers
1/2 tbsp. vegetable
   seasoning
1/2 tbsp. paprika
Grated soy cheese

Soak beans overnight with three times as much water. The next moarning rinse the beans, place in a pot with twice as much water, cover and bring to a boil. Reduce to simmer and simmer for about 35 minutes. If using carrots, dice into chunks and steam for 15 minutes.

Dice other vegetables and mix with Garbanzo beans and seasonings. Place in well buttered casserole dish, cover and bake at 325 degrees for 35 minutes. After 25 minutes put a layer of soy cheese on top.

THERESA'S ITALIAN SPAGHETTI

1 jar artichoke hearts,
   chopped
1/4 c. unrefined olive oil
4 or 5 cloves of garlic,
   minced
3 or 5 scallions, finely
   chopped

1 tsp. fresh basil, minced
1 pkg. DeBole's Jerusalem
   Artichoke substitute
   pasta (use fettucini or
   linguini)
or you may use fresh
   whole grain pasta
OR 1 pkg. Brown Rice
   noodles
OR 1 pkg. sesame noodles

For the noodles: Bring large saucepan of distilled water to a medium boil. While water is being heated, make sauce:

In small saucepan, on low heat, saute all the other ingredients in the Olive Oil, except the noodles. Stir and cook for about 10 minutes, being careful not to burn the garlic.

When water is boiling, add the noodles and cook for 4 to 5 minutes, or according to the package directions. Drain noodles and pour sauce over the noodles, quickly distributing it. You may add a pinch of cayenne pepper and/or sea salt if your diet allows. Serve with a tossed salad, or steamed vegetables. Enjoy!

JOHN'S MISO SAUCE FOR VEGETABLES

4 c. steamed root vegetables
2 tbsp. toasted sesame seeds
1 tsp. grated ginger root
1 tsp. minced garlic
2 tbsp. red miso

2 tsp. maple syrup
2 tbsp. dry sherry
1 tbsp. Chinese rice wine, optional
3 tbsp. lemon juice
2 tsp. roasted sesame oil

Combine all ingredients and toss with hot vegetables. Serve at once. Serves 4. This recipe also goes well over pasta.

MISO SOUP WITH VEGETATIAN DASHI STOCK

DASHI STOCK:

2 1/2 qts. water

3 inch piece of kombu seaweed

Boil kombu in water for 20 minutes. Strain out kombu and use remaining stock as follows (called dashi in following recipe).

MISO SOUP:

6 c. dashi
1/2 c. red miso
1/2 c. white miso
1 cake tofu, cut into small squares

1 scallion, minced
Tamari, to taste

Heat the stock to boiling, then remove 1 cup and mix with misos until smooth paste is formed. Return this to soup pot. Turn off heat. Drop in tofu and cover pot. Let sit 3 minutes. Pour into bowls and garnish with scallion and tamari. Serves 6.

CHILI SANS CARNE

1/4 c. olive oil
1 lg. green pepper, chopped
1 med. onion, chopped
4 cloves garlic, sliced
1 tsp. each salt and chili
    powder
1/2 c. bulghur wheat

2 c. cooked kidney or pinto
    beans (see over)
2 c. chopped tomato
1 tbsp. soy sauce
1 c. water

Heat oil in a good sized pot on medium heat. Saute onion for a few minutes, pepper a minute more, galric, salt and chili powder briefly, then add bulghur and stir a minute more. Add beans, tomato, soy sauce and water. Bring to a simmer, then reduce heat and simmer, covered, for at least 30 minutes, preferably longer, stirring occasionally. Makes 4 to 6 servings, freezes well, too.

VEGETABLE-TOFU STEW

1/2 c. oil Canola
1 lg. onion, sliced
1 or 2 cloves garlic, chopped
1 lb. tofu, cut into 3/4 inch
    cubes
2 med. carrots, sliced
1/4 head cabbage, chopped

1 summer squash or
    zucchini, chopped
1 c. water
1/3 to 1/2 c. soy sauce
    (Natural)
1 bay leaf
Pinch pepper

Heat oil in a good sized pot on medium heat. Saute onion for a few minutes, pepper a minute more, garlic, salt and chili powder briefly, then add bulghur and stir a minute more. Add beans, tomato, soy sauce and water. Bring to a simmer, then reduce heat and simmer, covered, for at least 30 minutes, preferably longer, stirring occasionally. Makes 4 to 6 servings, freezes well, too.

SCRAMBLED TOFU

1 lb. tofu, with moisture
   squeezed out
1 lg. sprig of parsley,
   minced (should equal
   about 1 tbsp.)
1 tsp. unrefined sesame oil
Pinch GOMASIO or sea salt

1/2 tsp. turmeric
1/2 tsp. cayenne pepper
2 tsp. sesame seeds,
   optional

Place Tofu in mixing bowl, mash well with fork. Add the turmeric and cayenne, mix well.

Heat medium sized skillet and add oil; flame should be moderate (not high!) When oil is hot (test by dropping tiny drop of water into skillet, it should evaporate immediately) add the parsley and saute for 2 minutes. Add the sesame seeds if desired, and the Gomosio seasoning. Stir well and then add the Tofu. Scramble (like eggs) for 2 to 3 minutes, until the Tofu is heated through. Remove from heat and serve with Whole Wheat tortillas or toasted Essene bread.

VARIATIONS:

Saute any of the following vegetables with the parsley:
Scallions, minced

peppers, chopped

black olives, sliced

Hijiki or Arame seaweed, soaked and drained

Minced garlic

You can also substitute the Turmeric with mexican seasonings such as Cilantro (minced), cumin, chili powder, etc., and serve with a Picante sauce or hot sauce. Try using fresh Dill or Basil in addition to the parsley.

Substitute the Turmeric with Curry powder, and for a spicier Scramble, add a few drops of Eden Hot Sesame Oil to the other oil when you are sauteeing.

Before adding the Tofu to the cooked vegetables, stir in 1 tablespoon of Tahini into the skillet, mix well. This makes a richer dish. This dish also is quite good cold, treat it like a spread or dip!

SEAWEED DELUXE

2 lg. onions, sliced thin
1/2 pkg. Hijuki seaweed
(rinse quickly in bowl,
then soak in distilled
water
until soft 20 minutes)
2 to 3 tbsp. Eden Hot
sesame oil (use more or
less to taste)

1 tbsp. Miso, optional
2 tbsp. brown rice vinegar
1/4 c. unrefined sesame oil
2 tsp. Kuzu (arrowroot)
optional

Heat the unrefined sesame oil in wok or skillet and saute the onions until soft. Add the hot oil, then add soaked seaweed including the liquid. Add Miso and Brown Rice Vinegar, stirring the Hijuki for 5 minutes. Put cover on for 7 to 10 minutes, stir again for 2 minutes, and add Kuzu (arrowroot) to thicken. Serve with Brown Rice.

Variations: Sautee the onions with eggplant and/or red bell pepper. Add sesame seeds. Then proceed as above.

SZECHUAN EGGPLANT

1 med. sized eggplant (1 1/2
lbs.)
2 tsp. salt
2 tsp. Tamari
3 to 4 lg. cloves garlic,
minced
2 to 3 scallions, chopped

2 tbsp. sesame oil
1/4 to 1/2 tsp. crushed red
pepper
Dash of wine or brandy
1 tsp. minced ginger root

Peel and cut eggplant into strips 1x2 1/2 inches. Sprinkle lightly with salt and let sit in a bowl 1/2 hour.

Heat oil in wok. When very hot, add garlic, ginger, stir fry about 30 seconds. Add scallions, cook 1 minute. Add the eggplant and red pepper, stir fry 30 seconds, turn heat down (low) and cover, cook for 15 minutes, stirring occasionally. The eggplant should be very tender, almost like a puree. Add liquor, Tamari and serve with brown rice.

VEGETABLE STROGANOFF

SAUCE:

8 oz. red bell peppers (net
    weight after removing
    seeds, etc.)
1 tbsp. Canola oil
1 tbsp. whole wheat flour

2 oz. Tofu, pressed
1/4 tsp. vegetable
    seasoning
1/4 tsp. paprika
3/4 c. (6 oz.) soy milk

Prepare the peppers, cut into thin strips, drop into boiling water, reduce to simmer for 10 minutes. Saute oil and stir in flour and milk slowly, bring to a "bubble".

Crumble tofu and stir into sauce until smooth. Add vegetable seasoning and paprika. Drain peppers and add to above.

VEGETABLES:

8 oz. squash
4 oz. zucchini
12 oz. carrots

8 oz. broccoli or
    cauliflower
4 oz. fresh peas

Slice carrots, squash and zucchini. Break broccoli or cauliflower into pieces. Place all vegetables except peas in a steamer pot, cover, bring to boil, reduce to simmer for 25 minutes. Add peas and steam for another 8 minutes.

STROGANOFF:

Remove steamed vegetables and place on individual plates. Pour sauce on top and serve on brown rice.

EXTRA RECIPES

Fabulous Desserts

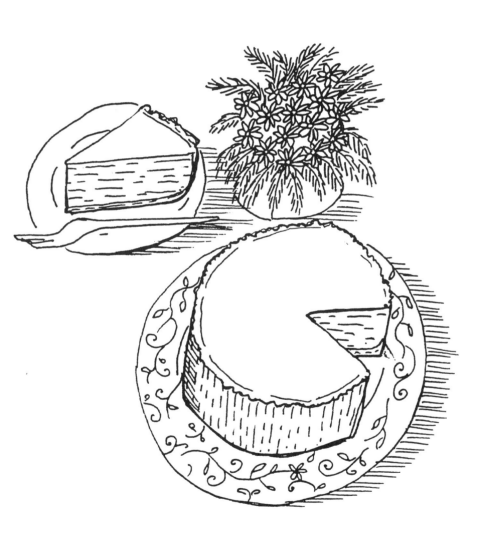

YUMMY CHEESECAKE

CRUST:

2/3 c. whole wheat flour
2 tbsp. honey
1/3 c. wheat germ
2 tsp. oil

1 egg yolks
2 tsp. water, if needed
Grated rind of one lemon

Blend all the ingredients together. Pat to cover bottom and sides of a 10 inch pan. Bake in a preheated 350 degree oven 5 minutes.

FILLING:

2 eggs plus 1 egg yolk
3 tbsp. yogurt cheese (kefir)
14 oz. tofu

1/4 c. honey
2 tbsp. lemon juice
1 tsp. vanilla
2 egg whites, beaten stiffly

Combine the two eggs plus yolk, kefir, tofu, honey, lemon juice and vanilla. Whirl the mixture in the blender or food processor until smooth. Fold in the egg whites. Pour the filling into the prepared crust and bake at 350 degrees 45 minutes, or until lightly browned. Let cool. Cake will fall as it cools.

PINEAPPLE TOPPING FOR CHEESECAKE

1 c. pineapple juice
1 tbsp. plus 1 tsp. agar
   flakes

2 c. crushed fresh
   pineapple

Heat the pineapple juice with the agar flakes to boiling. Stir a minute or two to dissolve. Let cook until thick but still liquid. Stir in the crushed pineapple. Using a slotted spoon, mount the pineapple onto the cooled cheesecake. Cool thoroughly before serving.

CREAMY TOFU PIE

2 lg. eggs or 1/3 c. vanilla
   soy milk
1/3 c. honey
1 lb. 6 oz. tofu
1 tsp. vanilla

2 tbsp. lemon juice
1 tsp. lemon peel

Put 1 egg and half the tofu and lemon juice (freshly squeezed) into a blender or food processor; cover and blend until smooth and creamy. Pour into a bowl; repeat with remaining egg, tofu and lemon juice. Stir in honey, vanilla and lemon peel.

Pour into a 9 inch pie shell or graham cracker crust. Bake 50 to 55 minutes, until a cake tester inserted in the middle comes out clean. Remove from oven and cool on a wire rack. Cover and chill three hours or longer.

PINEAPPLE TOPPING:

1 c. pineapple juice
1 tbsp. plus 1 tsp. agar
   flakes

2 c. crushed fresh
   pineapple

Heat the pineapple juice with the agar flakes to boiling. Stir a minute or two to dissolve. Let cook until thick but still liquid. Stir in the crushed pineapple. Using a slotted spoon mount the pineapple onto the cooled cheesecake. Cool thoroughly before serving.

Cathy Attal

ZUCCHINI BREAD

Beat three eggs until foamy. Add:

1 c. of safflower oil
3 tsp. vanilla

3/4 c. honey
3 c. grated squash

Sift:

3 c. rye flour
1 tsp. soda

1/4 tsp. baking powder
3 tsp. cinnamon

Mix together with first ingredients. Add 1 cup walnuts. Pour into oiled loaf pan. Bake 1 hour at 325 degrees or until done. Can be frozen.

PUMPKIN SPICE PIE

1 1/2 c. whole wheat pastry
    flour
1 1/2 c. brown rice flour
1/2 tsp. salt

1/2 c. safflower oil
4 to 6 tbsp. apple juice,
    cold

Sift flour and salt. Rub in oil until flour forms pea sized balls. Dribble cold juice over flour. Press with a fork, until dough forms one ball. Knead gently one minute to smooth texture. Divide dough in half. Refrigerate 1/2 hour. Roll out on wax paper 2 inches larger than pie pan. Fit crusts into two oiled, floured pie pans. Tuck overhanging edges in and crimp with fork or flute.

PIE FILLING:

6 to 8 cups pumpkin puree
    (vary with buttercup or
    butternut squash)
2 eggs, or 1/2 block soft
    tofu
1/4 c. arrowroot or kuzu
1/2 to 1 c. apple juice
1/4 to 1/2 c. maple syrup
    (or barley malt)

1/2 tsp. salt
2 tsp. cinnamon
2 tsp. nutmeg
1 tsp. cloves
1/2 tsp. ginger
1 c. roasted chopped
    walnuts

Wash one medium pumpkin; cut in half and remove seeds. Oil baking dish; pour 1/2 cup water into pan to cover bottom. Place pumpkin halves into dish, cut side down, cover with aluminum foil and bake at 375 degrees for 1 to 1 1/2 hours, until a fork easily pierces skin.

Dissolve arrowroot in 1/2 cup water or juice; blend with eggs (if substituting tofu, mix in blender), maple syrup, salt, spices. Pour egg mixture into bowl.

Cube cooked pumpkin (skin and all) and place in blender with egg mixture. Puree in batches. Add more juice if needed to blend puree. Fill 2 pie crusts. Bake at 350 degrees for 45 to 60 minutes. Pies should look set and may crack slightly. Garnish with walnuts. Allow to cool. This pie tastes best if made the day before. Makes 2 pies.

COCONUT BARS

1/2 c. safflower oil
   margarine (8 tbsp.)
1/2 c. barley-malt syrup
1 egg
2/3 c. brown rice flour
1 tsp. vanilla

1/2 tsp. baking powder
1 c. quick oatmeal
1 c. coconut
1/2 c. nuts, almond or
   walnuts

Cream margarine and barley-malt syrup together until light and fluffy. Add egg, blend. Add dry ingredients. Stir well, add oats, coconut, vanilla, nuts. Spread in greased 9x13 pan. Bake at 350 degrees for 20 to 25 minutes or until golden brown. Cut while warm, and cool before stacking. This makes a good lunch bag item.

NUTTY BANANAS

Mix 1/2 cup natural almond butter with 2 tbsp. soy milk. Peel two bananas, cut in half crosswise. Insert a stick in each flat end. Spread bananas with almond butter mixture and roll in chopped nuts. Place on waxed paper and freeze until firm, about 2 hours.

BANANA PUDDING

1 block tofu
3 ripe bananas
1 tbsp. lemon juice
1/4 tsp. salt

2 tsp. vanilla
1 tsp. almond extract
1/2 c. rice syrup
1/2 c. safflower oil

In blender whip all ingredients. Pour into pudding dishes, then chill overnight before serving.

CREME PIE

3 c. tofu
1 c. melted soy oil
   margarine
1/2 c. rice syrup

1/2 c. carob powder
2 tsp. vanilla
1/4 tsp. salt
1/2 c. tofu liquid

In blender, whip all ingredients, then pour into whole wheat pie crust and chill.

SWEET CUSTARD

Blend in blender:

1/4 c. whole wheat pastry
    flour
4 eggs
2 c. almonde #
    milk (see pag

1/4 c. honey
1/4 tsp. salt

Firmness of custard depends on ratio of eggs to milk. 1 egg per 1/2 cup of almond milk gives a soft baked custard. 325 degrees for 20 to 30 minutes.
1/2 tsp. of the following natural flavorings may be added to the custard: vanilla, rum, almond, orange extract or nutmeg.

BASIC CUSTARD

Beat together:

4 eggs
2 c. soy milk

1/2 tsp. salt
1/4 c. whole wheat flour,
    optional

Bake at 325 degrees for 20 to 30 minutes. 1/2 tsp. of the following natural flavorings may be added to the custard: vanilla, rum, almond, orange extract or nutmeg.

BAKED CUSTARD

1/4 c. rice flour
3 c. soy milk, scalded (or
    almond milk)
4 eggs

5 tbsp. honey
1/4 tsp. sea salt
1 tsp. pure vanilla
sprinkle with nutmeg

Pour all ingredients in blender (except nutmeg). Blend on blend cycle, then put in casserole dish or cups. Have a pan filled with hot water to set cups in. This recipe makes its own crust. Bake for 30 to 40 minutes at 350 degrees.

BLUEBERRY JELLY

Approximately 3/4 cup water to 2 lbs. berries. Cook until soft. Strain juice through jelly bag. Measure 1 cup juice, bring this to boiling point and add 1/4 cup honey and 1 tsp. lemon. Boil rapidly to jelly stage. Pour into sterilized glasses and seal.

BLUEBERRY JAM

Mash berries (not over ripe) and heat 1 cup berries through. Then add scant 1/4 cup honey, stir to desired consistency, pour into sterilized jars and seal while hot. Drain crushed pineapple (approximately 2 tsp to 1 cup jam) or both, can be added for additional flavor.

HIGH-PROTEIN DESSERT

1 tsp. tahini
1/2 c. plain yogurt (soy)
2 tbsp. walnuts

2 tbsp. raisins
Cinnamon to taste

Mix yogurt and Tahini together then sprinkle nuts and raisins over yogurt and tahini. Top with cinnamon. Easy, delicious and high in protein.

SUNNY BANANAS

1 tbsp. agar flakes, dissolve
   in cold water
1/2 c. boiling water, add and
   melt agar flakes
1 1/2 c. fresh carrot juice

3 very ripe bananas, sliced
1/2 c. dates, cut in small
   pieces

Set in refrigerator. Serve garnished with a little soy yogurt.

WHEAT GERM MUFFINS

1 c. whole wheat flour
1 tsp. salt
3 tsp. baking powder
1/4 c. powdered soy milk
1 c. wheat germ

1 c. soy milk
2 eggs
1/4 c. honey or molasses
2 tbsp. oil

Sift into mixing bowl the flour, salt, baking powder, and powdered soy milk. Add and stir only until moist the wheat germ, soy milk, honey or molasses, and oil.

Fill paper baking cups or well greased muffin pans two thirds full. Bake at 400 degrees for 15 to 20 minutes, or until brown. Makes a dozen large muffins.

NOTE: 1/2 cup raisins may be added with the wheat germ.

ORANGE SESAME MUFFINS

1 1/2 c. whole wheat flour
1/2 c. soy flour
1 tsp. salt
2 tsp. baking powder
1/4 c. whole sesame seeds

1 egg, beaten optional
1/2 c. almond milk
1/4 c. oil
1/2 c. honey
1 tbsp. organic orange peel

Mix together flours, salt, sesame seeds, and baking powder. In a separate bowl blend egg, almond milk, oil, and honey. Stir in orange peel. Pour this mixture into the dry ingredients and stir just enough to moisten them. Lumps are okay. Fill muffin wells two thirds full and bake at 375 degrees for about 20 minutes or until they are golden.

THERESA'S PIE CRUST

2 c. whole wheat pastry
   flour
3/4 c. soy oil margarine,
   slightly softened

1 tsp. salt
4 tbsp. ice water

Mix well, adding ice water a little at a time, using fork to insure mixture of ingredients. Flour cloth then put dough on cloth. Place Saran Wrap over ball of dough. Roll over Saran Wrap in even motions.

RYE FLOUR PASTRY CRUST

Sift together:

2 c. rye flour   **1/2 tsp. baking powder**

For a dessert crust, sprinkle a little cinnamon in with the flour. Cut in 2/3 cup soy margarine until dough looks like cornmeal. Add enough cold water to make a stiff dough. Don't stir too much. Divide into two or three pieces depending on how large pie pans are. Wrap with waxed paper and put into refrigerator to cool.

Treat this dough like pizza dough. It will fall apart if rolled out. Put piece of dough into middle of oiled pie pan. Push down with waxed paper. Sprinkle with a little rye flour to keep from sticking to your hands. Spread with fingers until pan is completely covered.

TOFU EGGLESS CARROT CAKE

1 lb. tofu
1 c. carrot juice
1/3 c. tahini
1 carrot, grated
1/2 c. date sugar (ground
    dates)
1/4 c. whole wheat flour

1 tbsp. orange rind
1 tsp. vanilla extract
1 tsp. almond extract
1/2 c. ground walnuts
soy oil margarine

Preheat oven to 350 degrees. Chop tofu, then add to blender and combine with carrot juice, tahini, grated carrot, date sugar, flour, orange rind, vanilla and almond extract. Blend well.

Prepare an eight inch springform pan by oiling with soy oil margarine and then coating the bottom and sides with ground walnuts. This is the crust.

Pour the batter into the prepared pan and bake for 40 minutes. The top will appear puffy and nearly black.

Remove from oven and refrigerate several hours before serving. Once the cake has cooled, the top will sink back down, forming a dark "crust".

To serve, remove springform rim and slide cake onto a serving plate.

CARROT TORTE

5 eggs
1 c. maple sugar*
1 tsp. grated orange rind
1 tsp. cinnamon
1 tsp. allspice
2 c. grated carrots
2 c. ground almonds or
    walnuts

1 tsp. almond extract or
    vanilla
1/2 c. whole wheat pastry
    flour
1 1/2 tsp. baking soda
1/2 tsp. cream of tartar
Soy margarine
Whole wheat flour for
    dusting pan

Separate the eggs into two mixing bowls; reserve the whites. Beat yolks with maple sugar until creamy. Add orange rind, allspice, grated carrots, ground nuts and almond extract or vanilla; beat well. Sift together flour and baking soda; add to yolk mixture, beat well. Reserve.

Preheat oven to 425 degrees. Add cream of tartar to egg whites and beat until stiff. Fold whites into yolk mixture until well distributed, but be careful not to overbeat (do not use an electric mixer).

Pour batter into a bundt pan that has been oiled with soy margarine and dusted with flour. Bake for about 50 minutes, or until a toothpick inserted in the center comes out clean.

Allow to cool completely, then turn from pan. Frost if desired with Seven Minute Frosting.

*NOTE: Maple sugar is pure maple syrup that has been granulated. It is available in health food stores or gourmet shops.

SEVEN MINUTE FROSTING:

2 egg whites
1/2 c. honey
1/4 tsp. cream of tartar,
    optional

1 tsp. almond extract
1 tsp. vanilla

Place all ingredients in a double boiler. While heating, beat constantly with a handheld electric mixer, at high speed, for seven minutes.

Frost cake immediately, then refrigerate before serving.

PEACE COOKIE

1 qt. coarsely chopped
    apples, with peels
1 c. water
1 c. brown rice flour
2 c. cornmeal
2 c. blended millet flour
5 1/2 c. whole wheat fine
    ground pastry flour
3 c. barley corn malt

1 c. toasted coconut
1/2 c. oil
2 tbsp. vanilla
2 tbsp. baking powder
Grated rind of one orange
Granted rind of one lemon
1/2 c. honey
2 tbsp. carob powder

Blend the apples and water. Mix all of the ingredients (except carob) for five minutes on medium blender speed. Reserve 1 1/2 cups of batter.

Spoon 1/4 cup of batter per cookie onto an oiled sheet pan. Optional: Add two tbsp. of carob powder to the reserved batter to make an icing. Use it to draw a peace symbol on each cookie. Bake in 350 degree oven for about 15 minutes or until done. Yield: 30 large cookies

HOLIDAY FRUIT CAKE (EGGLESS)

Fresh orange juice
2 lbs. dried pears
4 c. water
1 c. dried apricots
2 c. water
3 c. whole wheat pastry
    flour

1/2 tsp. salt
1/2 c. oil
1 c. walnuts, chopped
1 tsp. vanilla
1 orange rind, grated

Preheat oven to 350 degrees. Place pears and water in a saucepan and cover and simmer for 1/2 hour. Puree in blender. Place apricots and water in a saucepan. Cover and simmer for 1/2 hour. Chop. Combine flour and salt. Rub oil into the flour by hand. Add the pear puree, chopped apricots, walnuts, vanilla and orange rind to flour mixture. Add enough fresh orange juice to make a moist batter. Pour into a 9x5 inch pan. Bake 1 1/2 hours or until brown and a toothpick comes out clean. This cake keeps well in a refrigerator or in a freezer.

FRUITCAKE

If you think you don't like fruitcake, try this one - it's sure to change your mind, for it's chock full of real dried fruits instead of the bizarrely colored glazed bits used in most fruit cakes.

1 c. pitted dates, cut up
1 1/2 c. diced dried apples
1 c. dried apricot halves, cut in quarters
1 c. walnut halves

3/4 c. whole wheat flour
1/2 tsp. baking powder
1/4 tsp. salt
3 eggs
1/2 c. molasses
1 tsp. vanilla extract

Preheat oven to 300 degrees. Combine dried fruit and nuts. Combine flour, baking powder and salt, and add to dried fruit mixture. Stir well. Beat eggs, then beat in molasses and vanilla. Add to fruit mixture and stir until all ingredients are well moistened.

Spoon into a well greased 6 cup tube or ring mold. Bake for 1 hour. Cool in the pan for 10 minutes, then turn onto a rack and cool completely.

Makes 1 large ring.

NOTE: Fruitcake can be baked in a variety of pans, ranging from small muffin tins (baking time will be about 30 minutes) to an 8 inch loaf pan or square. To determine if the cake is done, insert a toothpick and, when it comes out clean, take the cake out of the oven. This cake stores very well, making it ideal for gift giving or mailing at holiday time. Wrap in foil to retain moistness.

PECAN PIE

FILLING:

1/2 c. dried apricots
1/2 c. dates, pitted
2 c. papaya juice
2 tbsp. agar flakes
Pinch of salt

1 1/2 tbsp. kuzu dissolved in 1/4 c. water
1 tsp. vanilla
2 c. roasted pecans

CRUST:

1 c. brown rice flour
1/2 c. whole wheat pastry
    flour
Pinch salt

1/4 c. oil (safflower)
3 to 4 tbsp. cold apple
    juice
Pinch of coriander or
    cardamom for extra
    flavor, optional

Rinse dried fruits, combine with juice, agar and salt in a saucepan. Bring to a boil, lower flame and simmer 20 minutes. Make crust, following directions. Crust must be pricked with a fork several times to prevent warping. Bake crust in 350 degree oven for 15 minutes or until light gold.

Pecans can be roasted at the same time, but watch them carefully, pecans burn easily after 10 minutes.

When the dried fruit is plump and agar is dissolved, add kuzu and stir until clear. Add vanilla. Puree fruit mixture in a blender or food processor until creamy smooth.

Save 1/2 cup of pecans to garnish top of pie. Mix the remaining pecans with the fruit puree. Spoon mixture into baked pie crust. Arrange 1/2 cup pecans in design on top of pie. Allow to cool. This pie should slice neatly and still be creamy.

Variations: This basic recipe can be adapted to your own tastes. Other types of dried fruit can be substituted. Filberts, walnuts or almonds can be used instead of pecans, and lemon or orange juice can be used for lighter flavor.

SWEET POTATO PIE

1 c. cooked mashed sweet
    potatoes
1/2 c. soy milk
1/3 c. melted soy or
    safflower margarine
2 beaten eggs

1 tsp. ground nutmeg
1/2 tsp. baking powder
1/2 c. honey
1 unbaked pie shell

Combine sweet potatoes with all ingredients except pie shell, blending well with electric mixer. Pour into pie shell. Bake in 400 degree oven for about 30 minutes or until golden and puffy.

FRUIT QUARTET

4 different kinds of dried
    fruit
Fresh orange slices
Water and/or fresh orange
    juice

Juice of one lemon
1 cinnamon stick

Combine fruits to your taste. Add several slices of fresh oranges, lemon juice and cinnamon stick. Cover the fruit with water and orange juice. Simmer until fruit is tender and sauce is thick. Serve for dessert or as an appetizer. Top with crushed walnuts or almonds.

DRIED FRUIT PIE

4 c. water
3 c. assorted dried fruits
2 tbsp. soy oil margarine

1/4 c. whole wheat flour
1 c. chopped nuts
1 partially baked whole
    wheat pie shell

Bring water and fruit to a boil. Reduce the heat and simmer until sauce is thick. Stir in margarine and flour. Remove from heat, and stir in chopped nuts. Blend half of mixture at a time in a blender. Pour into a partially baked pie shell, and bake for 20 minutes at 350 degrees. The pie looks like a dark molasses pie when done.

RICE PUDDING

1 c. brown rice
4 c. water
1/2 tsp. sea salt
1/4 c. tahini
1/2 c. raisins

2 eggs, lightly beaten or
    1/2 c. soy milk
2 tbsp. maple syrup
1/2 tsp. vanilla
1/4 tsp. cinnamon
2 pinches nutmeg

Wash rice thoroughly in cold water. Bring to a boil with a pinch of salt and 3 1/2 cups of the water and allow to boil for a few minutes; then reduce heat and simmer, covered, for 40 minutes. Dilute tahini with remaining 1/2 cup water, adding a little at a time and mixing until creamy.

In a covered baking dish combine rice, tahini, and all other ingredients except nutmeg, mixing well. Sprinkle nutmeg on top and bake at 350 degrees for 20 minutes, removing cover 5 minutes before done. Serves 6.

PUDDINGS AND PORRIDGE

If necessary, this pudding may be cooked entirely on top of the stove, just simmer on low heat instead of baking for the last 20 minutes. Simmered or baked, a variety of puddings can be prepared with rice or other whole grains or cereals. Use fresh or dried fruit, toasted seeds, or chopped nuts in place of, or in addition to, the ingredients given here, or use part apple juice for a different sweetness. A creamy breakfast porridge can be prepared by simmering rice in 4 to 5 parts water for 1 hour or more.

MAPLE SOY FROSTING

1 c. soy milk powder
1/2 c. maple syrup or rice
  syrup

2 tbsp. vanilla
3 tbsp. orange juice

Combine all ingredients and beat until smooth and creamy. Cake may be frosted and served immediately.

MAPLE CREAM FROSTING

8 oz. soy yogurt
1/2 c. maple syrup

1 tsp. vanilla

Beat all ingredients together until smooth and creamy. Frost cake immediately, then refrigerate before serving.

CAROB ICING

Cream together 2 tbsp. soy margarine, 2/3 cup sifted non instant powdered soy milk. Add the following in order: 1/3 cup toasted carob powder, 1/4 cup maple syrup (put maple syrup in saucepan with 1/8 cup water on medium flame, stirring constantly until it starts to thicken), 4 tbsp. soy milk, 1 tsp. vanilla, 1/2 tsp. almond extract.

Beat until smooth and spread on cake or brownies.

UNSWEETENED CAROB SYRUP

1 c. sifted carob powder   1 c. water

In a small saucepan, blend carob powder and water. Bring to a boil over very low heat, stirring constantly. Cook just under 10 minutes or until the syrup is smooth. Store covered in the refrigerator. Use in place of bitter or unsweetened chocolate, or as a sauce for deserts. Two tablespoons of soy margarine can be added, too.

SEMI-SWEETENED CAROB SYRUP

Follow recipe above but before simmering, add 1/4 cup honey (or to taste) plus 1 to 2 tablespoons unsalted safflower oil margarine.

SWEETENED CAROB SYRUP

1 c. sifted carob powder   1/4 c. barley malt syrup
1 tbsp. arrowroot   2 tsp. pure vanilla extract

Combine powder and arrowroot. Follow directions for unsweetened carob syrup above.

PEACH COBBLER

1 stick soy oil margarine   3/4 c. maple syrup
1 c. whole wheat pastry   (divided)
   flour   4 c. sliced peaches (fresh
1 c. soy milk   raw peaches sliced
                                     thinly)

Mix peaches with 1/2 cup of maple syrup and bring to a boil. Melt margarine in a 9x13x2 pan in a warm oven. Mix flour, remaining 1/4 cup maple syrup and soy milk in a bowl. Pour flour mixture over melted margarine. Pour hot cooked peaches evenly over flour mixture. Bake at 375 degrees for 30 minutes. A cake like crust forms on top and sides of pan. Serve hot.

WHEATLESS CARROT CAKE

2 c. of fine ground rice flour
2 tsp. baking soda
3/4 tsp. sea salt
1 c. maple syrup
1/3 c. oil (safflower)
2 eggs
1/4 c. liquid soy milk

2 tsp. lemon juice
3 med. carrots, grated
2 tsp. spices (cinnamon, cloves, nutmeg)
8 oz. fresh crushed pineapple
1/2 c. fresh shredded coconut

Oil a 10x10 pan and preheat the oven to 325 degrees. Sift the dry ingredients together and set aside. Mix maple syrup and oil well, until thick. Beat the eggs in, one at a time. Add the flour mixture to the maple syrup mixture in about three parts; after each addition, mix very well. Beat in liquid soy milk and the lemon juice. Stir in remaining ingredients, being sure they are evenly distributed throughout the batter. Place in pan and cook at 325 degrees for about 40 to 45 minutes or until evenly browned and a toothpick comes out clean. Please allow to cool 15 to 20 minutes before cutting.

A nice "icing" is: 1 c. of plain soy yogurt mixed with about 2 tbsp. of fresh lemon juice, this is just spooned on each serving of cake.

KIWIFRUIT COMPOTE

2 kiwifruit, pared and sliced
1 fresh pear, cored and cut into chunks
1 orange, peeled and sectioned
1 banana, peeled and sliced

1 c. red grapes, halved and seeded if necessary
1/2 tsp. grated orange peel
1/2 c. orange juice

Combine all ingredients except juice; spoon into fruit dishes or stemmed goblets. Pour liquid over mixture. Makes 4 to 6 servings.

MOLDED FRUIT DESSERT

1 c. water
1 c. apricot nectar
1/2 c. apple juice
1 tbsp. agar flakes
3 caffeine-free orange spice
    tea bags

1 c. strawberries, sliced
2 peaches, sliced
1 banana, sliced
1/2 c. blueberries, fresh or
    frozen

Bring water, apricot nectar, orange juice, lemon juice and agar to a boil. Reduce heat and simmer five minutes, stirring occasionally. Remove from heat, add tea bags, cover pan and let tea steep five minutes. Remove tea bags, pour mixture into a mold prerinsed with cold water, and refrigerate until mixture starts to set, about 20 minutes.

Meanwhile, prepare fruit. When agar mixture is ready, gently fold in fruit. Refrigerate until set. Unmold and garnish as desired. Serve plain or top with plain soy yogurt, whipped tofu topping, or natural vanilla or rice dream soybean ice cream.

OLD FASHIONED DANISH APPLE PIE

6 or 7 apples, peeled and
    sliced
3/4 c. barley-malt syrup or
    honey
1 stick of safflower oil
    margarine

1 1/2 c. whole wheat flour
A pinch of salt
1 tsp. cinnamon

First, oil a baking dish with safflower oil margarine. Place the apples in the dish and drizzle with barley-malt syrup or honey. Mix together margarine, flour, salt, and cinnamon. Sprinkle over apples and bake at 375 degrees for 45 minutes.

NOTE: Cut margarine in small pieces when mixing with flour, etc.

VEGAN O'CARROT CAKE

1/4 c. carrot juice
1 1/4 c. whole wheat pastry
   flour or brown rice flour
2 tsp. baking powder
1/2 c. maple syrup

2 tsp. cinnamon
1/4 c. wheat germ,
   optional
1 c. grated carrots
1/2 c. raisins
1/2 c. chopped walnuts

Preheat oven to 350 degrees. Blend the carrot juice with 1/4 cup of the flour, 1 tsp. of the baking powder, and 1 tsp. of the oil. Add the maple syrup. Reserve.

Sift the remaining cup of flour and tsp. of baking powder together with cinnamon, then add the wheat germ. Add to the maple syrup mixture with the remaining oil. Add the carrots, then fold in the raisins and walnuts.

Pour into a lightly greased nine by nine inch pan and bake for 30 to 40 minutes. Cool slightly before serving.

DRIED FRUIT MUNCHIES

1 c. dates, ground in meat
   grinder
1 c. in
   dried apricots, ground
1 c. dried pears, ground in
   meat grinder

1 c. dried apples, ground in
   meat grinder
2 tbsp. lemon rind, grated
   fine
1/2 c. chopped nuts,
   optional

Work all ingredients together by hand. Shape into balls. Roll in chopped nuts or in shredded coconut.

PIE CRUST

3 oz. raisins, ground fine
3 oz. walnuts or brazil nuts,
   ground fine

1/2 c. shredded coconut
1 tbsp. lemon rind, grated
   fine

Work together with hands into a pliable dough. Press into pie dish.

PIE FILLINGS:

Persimmons, peeled and sliced. Apples, sliced. Bananas, sliced 1 tsp. lemon rind, grated fine, 3 tbsp. fresh, shredded coconut. Whipped papaya sprinkled with shredded coconut. Sliced bananas. Fresh strawberries, creamed.

ALMOND BUTTER-DATE SPREAD

1/2 c. dates	2 tbsp. coconut
1/2 c. water	1 tbsp. lemon juice
1/2 c. almond butter	

Simmer dates in water until soft. Add rest of ingredients and mix well.

FRENCH CAROB MOUSSE

4 egg yolks	1 tsp. vanilla
1/2 c. carob powder	4 egg whites
1/3 c. soy milk	

Blend the egg yolks, carob, milk and vanilla for about 30 seconds at low speed. In a bowl, beat the egg whites until quite stiff. Fold the blender mixture into the whites and spoon into 5 or 6 cups. Set in the refrigerator or eat at once. Serves 5 or 6.

Total of approximately 40 calories each serving. You may add 2 tablespoons honey to the egg yolks, carob, soy milk and vanilla.

CARROT BREAD PUDDING

3 to 4 cups leftover carrot cake, cubed	3 eggs
1/2 c. raisins	1/3 c. honey
1/2 c. chopped or ground nuts	1 tbsp. vanilla
8 oz. tofu	1 tbsp. cinnamon
1 soft banana, mashed	3 c. milk "soy"
2 apples, grated with skins	

Preheat oven to 350 degrees. Lightly grease a 9x13 inch baking pan and spread evenly with carrot cake cubes. sprinkle with raisins and nuts. Reserve.

In blender, combine tofu, banana, apples, eggs, honey, vanilla and cinnamon. Blend well, then add enough milk to make 4 to 5 cups of liquid (depending on how many cups of leftover carrot cake you have). Liquify. Pour liquid over the cake, raisins and nuts in the pan. Bake for 35 minutes. Serve hot or cold.

WHOLE WHEAT FLOUR CREPES

1 c. yogurt	**2/3 c. whole wheat flour**
3 eggs	**1/4 c. water**

Mix all ingredients until smooth and let stand 30 minutes. If batter is too thick, add a little more water. It should have the consistency of heavy cream or buttermilk.

Wipe a 7 inch skillet with oil over moderate heat. Add a scant quarter cup of batter to the skillet and tilt it quickly to cover the bottom with batter. If the batter is too thick, it won't run fast enough. Any "holes" left in the pan can be patched with a drop of the batter. Cook until the edges appear dry and the batter is set in the center. Lift the crepe gently with a spatula and set aside. Repeat until all the batter is used. Makes about 12 crepes.

NOTE: Wiping the pan with oil ensures a non stick surface. Excess oil produces a lacy, fragil crepe that will fall apart.

Swirling the batter in the pan takes only a bit of practice. Right handed beginners might try pouring batter with the left hand while tilting the pan with the right. Lefties do the opposite.

Crepes are cooked on one side only. Unused crepes may be frozen in a stack, well wrapped with paper between the layers.

FILLINGS:

Sauteed vegetables such as onion, bell pepper, squash, eggplant, carrots. Chopped fruit such as fresh pineapple, peaches, strawberries. Sauteed nuts, black olives, and spinach.

FRUIT "FONDUE"

Fresh fruits cut in bite size pieces (berries, seedless grapes, pitted cherries, peaches, cantaloupe, etc.
HONEY-YOGURT DRESSING:
Put dressing in a bowl in the center of a large platter. Arrange fruits around it. Serve with fondu forks to dip fruits in the dressing.

AMBROSIA

1 c. chopped pineapple
1 c. orange sections

4 tbsp. unsweetened shredded coconut

Gently toss together the pineapple and the orange sections. Spoon into four small dessert dishes. Sprinkle 1 tablespoon of the coconut over each. Serves 4.

SPROUTED MUESLI

1/2 c. sesame seeds
1/2 c. sunflower seeds
1/2 c. chopped dates

1/2 c. chopped dried apples
1/2 c. raisins or currants
1/2 c. sprouted wheat, ground

Blend first two ingredients to a fine meal. Mix in a bowl with last 4 ingredients. To serve, moisten with apple juice or almond milk.

NUT AND SEED MILK 1

1/2 c. almonds, blanched
1/2 c. sesame seeds or cashews

1 qt. water
2 tbsp. rice or barley malt syrup

In an electric blender or food processor, blend ingredients until smooth.

NUT AND SEED MILK II

1/2 c. sunflower seeds   1/4 c. almonds
1/4 c. walnuts   1 c. pure water

    In an electric blender or food processor, blend ingredients until smooth.

ALMOND MILK

1 c. almonds, blanched   2 tbsp. barley malt syrup
1 qt. pure water   1/4 tsp. lecithin (optional,
                                          this makes a creamier
                                          milk)

    Pour a cup of boiling water over the almonds and let stand for 3 minutes to blanch them, this softens the skins and the meat. In an electric blender or food processor, blend ingredients until smooth. Also good as a hot drink.

SESAME CREAM

5 oz. sesame seeds   4 oz. water
4 oz. honey or barley malt
    sweetener

    Grind sesame seeds in nut grinder. Blend water and honey and gradually add ground sesame seeds. Chill before serving. Excellent on desserts and fruit salads. Makes 1 1/2 cups.

Breads

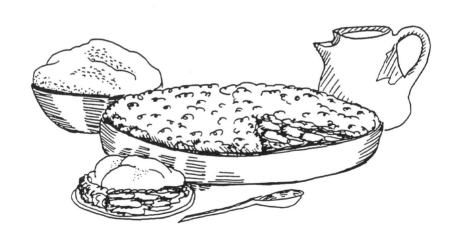

SPROUTED GRAIN CRACKERS

1/2 c. sprouted wheat
1 c. sprouted rye
1 tsp. caraway seeds,
   powdered

1 tsp. kelp
1/2 tsp. onion powder

Grind sprouted grains in meat grinder three times. Add remaining ingredients. Work into a pliable dough. Dust cutting board with arrowroot powder. Roll out dough to 1/8 inch thickness. Cut into squares. Place on rack. Cover with cheese cloth. Put outside in direct sun and dry to desired hardness.

Serving suggestions: Cream one avocado with 1/2 tsp. onion powder. Spread mixture on crackers, sprinkle sprouted sesame seeds on top.

ZUCCHINI BREAD

3 eggs
2/3 c. oil
2/3 c. honey
3 tsp. vanilla
3 c. grated squash

3 c. rye flour
1 tsp. soda
1/4 tsp. baking powder
3 tsp. cinnamon
1 c. chopped walnuts

Beat the eggs until foamy. Add the oil, honey, vanilla, and squash. In separate bowl, sift 3 cups rye flour, soda, baking powder and cinnamon. Mix together with first ingredients. Add nuts.

Bake one hour at 325 degrees until done. Should make one loaf pan and one 8x8 cake pan.

Cathy Attal

RYE DATE SQUARES

1/2 c. rye flour
1/2 c. rolled oats
1 c. chopped nuts
1/2 tsp. baking powder
1 c. date pieces

2 eggs or 1/3 c. soy milk
1/2 c. honey
1/3 c. oil
1/2 tsp. vanilla

Mix in a small bowl the flour, oats, nuts, baking powder and date pieces. In a mixing bowl combine the eggs, honey, oil, and vanilla. Beat until creamy and smooth. Add slowly to dry ingredients and stir well. Pour into well greased 9x12 pan and bake at 350 degrees for approximately 30 to 35 minutes. Let cool and cut into squares.

Cathy Attal

RICE FLOUR MUFFINS

1 c. rice flour
2 tsp. baking powder
Pinch of salt
1/2 c. ground oats
1/4 c. honey
1/4 c. sesame oil

1 c. soy milk
2 eggs
1/4 c. nuts, ground
1/2 c. raisins or fresh
   blueberries

Combine all dry ingredients in one bowl. Mix wet ingredients in another bowl. Lightly oil and flour a 12 hole muffin tin. Preheat oven to 425 degrees. Mix contents of two bowls and spoon into muffin tins. Place in oven and bake for 20 minutes.

COUNTRY CORNBREAD

1 c. whole wheat flour
3/4 c. yellow cornmeal
2 tsp. baking powder
1/2 tsp. sea salt

2 tbsp. honey
1 egg, beaten
2/3 c. yogurt (soy)
1/4 c. oil

Heat oven to 425 degrees. Oil an 8x8x2 pan. Stir the dry ingredients together. Stir the liquid ingredients together and blend into the dry ingredients. Stir just to blend, do not overmix. Bake at 425 degrees for 20 to 25 minutes.

SOUTHERN STYLE BISCUITS

2 c. whole wheat flour
2 1/2 tsp. baking powder
1/2 tsp. salt

1/2 tsp. baking soda
1/3 c. soy margarine
3/4 c. yogurt (soy)

Sift the dry ingredients into a mixing bowl. Cut in the margarine. Stir in the yogurt and blend until it just holds together.

Remove to a floured board and knead for 1 to 2 minutes. Do not overknead. Roll out in a circle about 1/2 inch thick. Cut the biscuits with a floured biscuit cutter. Before placing on baking sheet, dip into additional melted margarine. Bake at 450 degrees for 10 to 12 minutes.

NOTE: For high, fluffy biscuits, the dough should be 1/2 to 3/4 inch thick. For thin, crusty biscuits it should be 1/4 inch thick.

For STRAWBERRY SHORTCAKE add 1 to 2 tbsp. honey to the yogurt. Bake as directed. Cut the hot biscuits in half and spoon chopped strawberries onto them. Other berries or peaches can also be used.

EXTRA RECIPES

INDEX

Fabulous Desserts

Salads, Dressings and Gravy

Soups